# PRACTICAL AROMATHERAPY

*How to Use Essential Oils to Restore Vitality*

**Shirley Price**

Thorsons

Thorsons
*An Imprint of* HarperCollins*Publishers*
77–85 Fulham Palace Road,
Hammersmith, London W6 8JB

The Thorsons website address is: www.thorsons.com

First published by Thorsons 1983
Second edition, fully revised 1987
Third edition, 1994
This revised and updated edition, 1999

4 6 8 10 9 7 5

A catalogue record for this book
is available from the British Library

ISBN 0 7225 3906 1

Printed and bound in Great Britain by
Omnia Books Limited, Glasgow

# CONTENTS

| | | |
|---|---|---|
| *Acknowledgements* | | vii |
| *Introduction* | | ix |
| *Chapter one* | AROMATHERAPY AND YOU | 1 |
| *Chapter two* | ESSENTIAL OILS | 7 |
| *Chapter three* | THE SKIN | 16 |
| *Chapter four* | COMPLEMENTARY THERAPIES AND HOLISM | 31 |
| *Chapter five* | SWISS REFLEX THERAPY (SRT) | 53 |
| *Chapter six* | SIMPLE AROMATHERAPY TREATMENT TECHNIQUES | 73 |
| *Chapter seven* | AN EXPLANATION OF MASSAGE | 82 |
| *Chapter eight* | AROMATHERAPY MASSAGE TECHNIQUES | 87 |
| *Chapter nine* | PREPARING OILS FOR MASSAGE | 114 |
| *Chapter ten* | RECIPES | 120 |
| *Chapter eleven* | TABLE OF ESSENTIAL OILS | 133 |
| *Chapter twelve* | THERAPEUTIC INDEX | 182 |
| *Chapter thirteen* | CASE HISTORIES | 197 |
| *Useful Addresses* | | 216 |
| *Index* | | 222 |

# ACKNOWLEDGEMENTS

I would like to thank my husband Len, without whose patience and consideration this book would never have been written.

## AUTHOR'S NOTE

Reference is made in this book to the internal use of essential oils. Many people do use essential oils internally, and with great success. Therefore this book does give guidelines to the correct dosage (for added safety for those people wishing to use this therapy). The decision whether to use essential oils internally must be at the discretion of the individual.

In the opinion of the author, essential oils should only be taken internally under the guidance of an aromatherapist who has continued training for a further two years on an aromatology course accredited by the Institute of Aromatic Medicine (see Useful Addresses).

N.B. It is imperative for any aspect of aromatherapy that only pure and natural essential oils from a reputable supplier are employed, and not perfume fragrances or synthetic fragrances.

# INTRODUCTION

Aromatherapy is a treatment designed to help maintain good health by the correct use and application of essential oils obtained from plants. The word 'aroma' means a fragrance or sweet smell, a subtle pervasive quality, the fragrance in plants, spices and other substances, and 'therapy' means a treatment designed to cure.

As the fragrance in a plant *is* its essential oil it is easy to see that aromatherapy is a treatment using essential oils. But knowing what aromatherapy is is only the beginning. In order to understand thoroughly the full meaning it is necessary first to discover and learn about the origins and power of essential oils themselves, and then to learn the various methods by which the oils can be used effectively.

## WHAT ARE ESSENTIAL OILS?

Every living thing has a life force, energy or 'soul' which it is impossible to get hold of or to see. It is this life force which, in human beings, is so wonderful and awe aspiring when we stop to consider the amazing facts about our bodies. It is this life force which is there even when our bodies are in poor health, giving us the strength to try and regain normal health.

The 'life force' of a plant is also something that cannot be seen or touched, and it has been said that it is contained in the essential oil of a living plant. It is the 'heart' of a plant and is present in only very, very small quantities, sometimes as little as .01 per cent. It is the energy from the original life force of the plant which we introduce into the body by aromatherapy, each oil having its own curative effect on certain parts of the body and its systems as well as greatly influencing the mind.

It has been said that essential oils are actually the 'hormones' of the plants. This is easy to believe, because the hormones *we* produce during our whole lifetime, and without which we cannot live, are present in very, very small quantities also, and would only fill a thimble! Similarly, it would take at least ten large buckets full of orange blossoms to extract a mere thimbleful of neroli essential oil. As our glands produce various hormones which affect our bodily systems, so the plant 'hormones' are capable of giving different effects, when used correctly.

Actually hormones (from the Greek *hormaein*, meaning 'to impel') are produced by our apocrine glands to impel, or stir up, a reaction in ourselves. I believe essential oils may also be like human pheromones (from the Greek *pherein*, 'to bear', together with hormone), which are the chemicals responsible for our personal 'smell'. Pheromones are produced (also in small quantities) by our apocrine glands, but this time to produce a reaction in others, as in sexual attraction (or the reverse!) The essential oils produced by plants certainly stir up reactions in human beings!

Because of this seemingly mystical quality, many people in this century were sceptical about the medicinal effects of plant oils. But, apart from the known facts of history, when plants and their essences were the only available remedies for disease, a lot of research has been conducted recently by doctors and chemists, and the results have shown that the ancients knew what they were doing!

Research has also unearthed some of the hazards which may present themselves if certain essential oils are mis-used, i.e. used neat or in strong concentrations over a long period of time. However, when used as recommended, in a sensible way, the hazards are few. In aromatherapy only a few *drops* of oil are used; to have an adverse effect a few teaspoonfuls would be needed. If discussing the possible hazards of smoking, it is like comparing the lungs of a person who smokes 1 cigarette a week with one who smokes 30 cigarettes a day. 'All things are poison – nothing is poison.' (Paracelsus)

## THE BACKGROUND OF AROMATHERAPY

The history of the use of aromatic oils on the body goes back at least 2,000 years before Christ. There are records in the Bible of the use of plants and their oils, both in the treatment of illness and for religious purposes. The Egyptians used them widely, both as cosmetics and for embalming their dead in order to delay decomposition. They were known in China perhaps even before that time, then their use gradually spread to the Greeks and Romans, who of course brought the idea to Britain.

The earliest written record of their use in England was in the thirteenth century, and from that time a great increase was shown in both oils produced and treatments carried out. Glove makers used to perfume their gloves with essential oils to mask the body odour of the wearer, and it was a known fact that, in the Middle Ages, in times of cholera and other diseases, the perfumers very rarely succumbed to illness. This was because nearly all essential oils are good antiseptics. Nicholas Culpeper's book on herbs, originally written in

1652 and recently reprinted, contains detailed properties of hundreds of medicinal plants.

However, in the nineteenth century, chemists began to produce chemical copies of essential oils; much cheaper to make and effective, though as perfumes, not as treatments. There then followed experiments with chemicals to try and imitate the medicinal properties of the oils, and gradually these were so successful that plants and their therapeutic qualities were in danger of becoming extinct.

Nevertheless, the early twentieth century brought a renewed interest in natural products and treatments, perhaps because many of the synthetic drugs had unwanted side effects. Nowadays true essential oils, which have practically no drawbacks when properly employed, are used extensively in the natural health field to improve and maintain health.

A chemist called Gattefossé, who wrote the first modern book on aromatherapy (indeed, he coined the word) discovered, after seriously burning his hand in his laboratory, that lavender was a wonderful healer of burns. His hand healed in a very short time, leaving no scar. He experimented on soldiers' wounds during World War I and discovered oils which greatly accelerated the healing process.

His work revealed that it was possible for essential oils to penetrate the skin and, via the extra-cellular liquids, reach the blood and lymph, which in turn carried them in the circulation to the organs. This whole process varies in each individual and with each oil, taking as little as half an hour in some people and as long as 12 hours in others. Actual skin penetration takes only a matter of minutes.

Dr Jean Valnet, a French physician, also experimented with essential oils and treated many of his patients by this method. His book on aromatherapy is well-known and respected. One of his favourite treatments was the use of essential oils in compresses on the affected part, because of the great penetrative powers which the oils possess. He once treated a young adult who had scars from a scald in his childhood by this method, and the scars reduced so considerably after several treatments that they were hardly noticeable.

Madame Maury, who died a few years ago (and whose husband was a notable homeopath) was interested in beauty therapy and natural medicines. She also carried out research with essential oils, and developed the massage techniques of aromatherapy, leaving the internal and other methods of use to naturopathic doctors.

She was eventually persuaded to come to England, where she set up an aromatherapy clinic in London. She also taught the subject, and through Madame Maury passing on her knowledge, mainly to beauty therapists, many now practise aromatherapy and several eminent people teach the subject. Their pupils nowadays are not only beauty therapists but also include a wide variety of health practitioners: acupuncturists, osteopaths, nurses, physiotherapists, reflexologists, medical herbalists and also orthodox doctors who are looking to avoid prescribing drugs to treat the side-effects of allopathic treatment.

# chapter one

# AROMATHERAPY AND YOU

In ancient times, in the East, people visited their 'physician' not when they were ill, but when they were *well*. If they became ill just after the visit and the physician hadn't foreseen the illness, they didn't pay the bill! Physicians were then mainly acupuncturists, and *kept* the bodily systems in health by regular treatment of all the pressure points on the body, thus ensuring good blood and lymph circulation.

This theory still holds good. If we could keep our blood circulating freely, and the lymph moving at its correct speed round the body, illness would be greatly reduced.

But how many of us have a perfect circulatory system? And why not?

Because, somehow, we all manage to produce tension of some sort in our bodies, either physical or emotional. Not only does modern living lessen the amount of exercise we give our muscles, but we sit with our spines bent, we walk incorrectly, and when we stand we let our weight go first on one leg and then the other.

The effect of this is that our muscles are working overtime to keep us in our 'slovenly' positions; tissues and organs are pushed into the wrong place, pressure is applied where it shouldn't be, and the result is that the blood and lymph have greater difficulty in flowing round evenly, and the toxins and waste carried by the venous and lymphatic systems cannot be eliminated quickly enough by natural means, so therefore they escape into the tissues, causing disturbances in the bodily systems and organs.

The emotional tensions we suffer bring much more serious consequences. Heart and blood pressure symptoms, sometimes due to incorrect diet, are more often brought about by tension due to things such as traffic (this affects us more than is realized if it is a daily double trip through a large city) or the pressure of work, or the day to day worries which some people cannot seem able to deal with in a relaxed manner.

The other effect on the blood circulation is simply the ageing process. In youth, while we are growing, the body cells are constantly dying and being renewed in every single part of the body; every cell of every bone, muscle, nerve and every drop of blood is continually being replaced, therefore all the organs, including the skin, go through this never-ending process of renewal.

As we get older, the dead cells take longer to be thrown off and longer then to be absorbed (or rejected – in the case of skin) and the new cells take longer to form and grow. This slowing down of the regeneration of cell tissue shows itself by a slowing down of all bodily functions, loss of energy, possible constipation, muscles without good tone, loose and often sallow skin.

It is now generally accepted that our state of mind can affect the health of our body, and many illnesses today have a psychosomatic origin. The mind is the most important part of us, yet it is the one thing we cannot touch or even X-ray. It is responsible for our feelings: love, hate, generosity, selfishness, anger, fear, embarrassment, frustration – what a long list of components there are that make up the mind.

Essential oils have much the same effect on us, except that they have first to be chosen to suit the emotional upset, and then be applied and hence absorbed into the bloodstream.

If the art of relaxation can be practised, whether by yoga, mind dynamics or by hypnotherapy, then the mind itself can be strengthened in positive application, and a better life can be lived by the owner of that mind, positively affecting both career and health.

Given belief in ourselves, practically anything is possible; it is known that *determination* to succeed is almost inevitably followed by success, in just the same way that determination not to succumb to the common cold will almost inevitably send it away with only the mildest of symptoms. It is no use trying to help someone who does not believe in the method of help used, because their mind has automatically put up a negative barrier.

People already convinced about natural products are more prepared to believe that brown bread is better for health than white bread than someone who thinks health food eaters are just cranks; bread is just bread and white tastes better anyway!

By making a conscious effort at a quiet time each day to relax, and train our minds to run only in *positive* channels leading to success and health, we can greatly minimize the negative channels, which only lead to physical and mental disease.

Finally, the other aspect of living which affects our bodily and mental health is our *diet*. Eating a lot of artificially prepared foods containing chemical additives is not conducive to good health or clear skin. The skin reflects the condition of the body, which in turn gives us an idea of the state of mind. No skin preparations, natural or otherwise, will improve the texture or appearance of a blemished skin so long as unsuitable foods are continually being eaten.

Unnatural (i.e., refined and artificially processed) foods, including white sugar, are a contributory factor to ill-health, as much as physical and mental stress. With this type of diet we are putting the digestive system under tension; too many rich foods can lead to troubles in the gall bladder or stomach.

Overconsumption of sugar (white, refined) and animal fat is often said to contribute to heart disease. The organs of elimination become congested because too many refined starchy foods are eaten, with not enough roughage, and this in itself can cause malfunctions within our systems.

What a sad story!!

However, all these harmful effects can be considerably minimized if we can keep our blood circulation as healthy as possible. Unaided we can see that we eat only the correct foods and not too much of them! (The high-fibre diet is an excellent example of giving the roughage needed to keep the bodily systems in good order, and one can eat a lot yet lose weight with this diet, too!)

When the mind is at peace, we experience only positive feelings like love, contentment, selflessness, generosity, etc., and our body responds by being healthy. At other times anger, fear, jealousy, selfishness and depression dominate, and these adversely affect the state of the body. Hormones are released automatically to cope with these feelings and try to return them to a positive state as quickly as possible.

We can make sure that we not only get plenty of exercise, but also re-educate ourselves in the art of sitting, standing and moving correctly. The trouble is that these things need a conscious effort of will, and we have to be really keen and interested to persevere until it simply becomes a habit.

Nonetheless, there is another way to help ourselves, and this is by the use of essential oils.

We tend to wait these days until we are showing symptoms of illness before going to be treated, whereas prevention is, and always will be, better than the cure. Aromatherapy is a very good way of *keeping* healthy, and should be used as a preventative treatment in the same way as the Chinese used acupuncture centuries ago.

Methods of getting essential oils into the blood stream (other than by taking them internally) are by baths, inhalations, compresses and various types of massage, varying from simple effleurage through to more advanced forms such as lymph drainage, neuro-muscular technique and shiatsu (where the acupressure points on the meridian lines are used).

## AROMATHERAPY BODY MASSAGE

Regular aromatherapy treatments from a qualified person will bring about, and retain for much longer, a dramatic improvement in well-being and general health, increased vitality and a visible improvement in the texture and colour of the skin.

Every treatment is individual – no two people are exactly the same, and many factors must be taken into consideration when deciding on the form the treatment will take, and the oils that will be used.

Essential oils are extremely concentrated. One drop in 10 to 20ml of carrier oil will give an identifying aroma, and in fact the true aroma of the plant is obtained by the correct dilution of the essence. Essential oils in their natural state give off too strong an aroma to be pleasant, and this is an important fact to consider. Each one gives off its own particular waves, affecting different people in various ways. From the nose a message is sent to the brain, and either pleasure or distaste results as the brain interprets the message.

Our olfactory nerves play a very big part in the success of the treatment, so the oils chosen must, when blended in the carrier oil, have an aroma that is pleasing. If the person does not like the fragrance it is necessary to find other oils which have the same therapeutic effect but are more appealing aesthetically.

A good aromatherapist will blend oils, taking into consideration the volatility, the effects on the bodily or mental conditions, and also the effect of the aroma on the person being treated. This last, as mentioned earlier, is of equal importance to the other two, when essential oils are being used in a specialized aromatherapy massage.

It is important, and interesting, to note that after an aromatherapy massage a bath or shower should not be taken until three to four hours after treatment, to ensure full absorption of the essential oils (even though they appear to have penetrated fully).

Should there not be an aromatherapist in your area it is possible to help yourself at home by using essential oils in various ways, all of which will be dealt with in detail in the following chapters.

# chapter two

# ESSENTIAL OILS

Much has been said about essential oils so far, but without mentioning how they are obtained, what the various oils will do or how the oils themselves vary in quality. Only oils obtained by steam distillation and expression can be truly classed as essential oils; those obtained by using some kind of solvent are known as absolutes or resins. These, even though the same part of a plant may be used as for distillation, yield an oil containing very different constituents and therefore having a completely different aroma, for example rose oil. The oil obtained from the distilled petals contains all plant constituents which are highly volatile, the resulting oil (which is practically colourless) being called either rose oil or rose otto. (In this book I have used the word 'otto' whenever I am referring to the distilled oil.) The oil obtained from solvent extraction is always referred to as rose absolute. All absolute and resinoid oils contain only the plant constituents which are soluble in the solvent used, which means that some heavier constituents are also included, such as those which make up the colour of the plant.

Distilled oils are considered to be the best for therapeutic use, the absolutes being indispensable to the perfume industry, for whom it is the *aroma* which is of paramount importance, whether synthetic or natural.

Earlier, the mystical quality of essential oils was mentioned – the energy of the plant. This quality varies during each day or season, and this naturally affects the oil itself. The explanation for this is that during the life of the plant the essential oil cells (distributed throughout the leaves, flowers, stems, bark or root in minute odiferous droplets) change their chemical composition according to the time of day or the season of the year.

It is therefore important to gather herbs and plants for therapeutic use, or distillation into essential oils, at exactly the right time – not so easy in these days of regular working hours!

The time for harvesting is dependent upon many things and lavender contains its highest percentage of oil between 10 a.m. and 4 p.m., making harvesting a very warm job, to say the least, as it is harvested in late July or early August!

Ylang-ylang blossoms all the year round, but the May and June flowers yield the highest percentage of essential oils.

The amount of oil present in plants varies considerably; in some it is as little as .01 per cent, which makes the resultant concentrate very expensive; in some it is as much as 10 per cent, which results in a reasonably priced oil.

A producer of essential oils has to take into consideration loss of oil by evaporation once the plant is picked and is being transported to the distillery. In the east they still distill lemongrass and one or two other grasses on the spot, usually in a portable copper still which they set up by the stream where the plants are growing. This way they get maximum oil yield.

Other factors which influence the quality and yield of essential oil in a plant are the different soil conditions in which they are grown and the variations in climate of different countries;

e.g., French lavender, English peppermint and Bulgarian rose otto are the most expensive oils of their type.

Essential oils are usually secreted from special glands, ducts or cells in one or several parts of aromatic plants, and from the sap and tissues of certain trees. They are present in the roots, stems, barks, leaves and/or flowers in varying quantities, and in certain botanical families they are more abundant than in others, for example:

Coniferae –     which speaks for itself; it includes all pines and cypress trees

Myrtaceae –     which family includes eucalyptus, and

Lamiaceae –     to which all mints belong, and which has among its members the useful aromatic plants of lavender, peppermint and rosemary.

The more oil glands or ducts present in the plant, the cheaper the final cost of the oil, and oils from plants with few oil producing glands are necessarily more expensive, for example:

100 kilos of eucalyptus yields about 4 litres oil.

100 kilos of some varieties of lavender oil can yield almost 1.5 litres oil.

100 kilos of some varieties of rose petals can give a yield of up to 20ml oil.

So we discover that the cost of producing essential oils is not only in direct proportion to the quality of the plant, as stated earlier, but is also dependent on the quantity of oil-producing glands present in the plant.

An essential oil can be made up of many separate substances, and those from flowers are much more complicated than those from leaves - the former may have more than one hundred components while some leaf essential oils may have only a few.

Aromatherapists use them in their natural 'mixed' state, when they have a powerful synergy (the working together) of all the components of a 'whole' oil.

Chemists can break down an essential oil into its separate components of terpenes, esters, ketnones etc., of which it is composed, and extract the part they want to use; for example, thymol is taken from thyme essential oil, and menthol is taken from peppermint essential oil. We are familiar with both these substances in present day medicine, but probably did not realize that they were from the actual essential oil produced from a plant.

**Note:** In general the more an essential oil is interfered with chemically or physically the more its therapeutic powers are diluted — and the more likely there are to be side effects.

The strength at which an essential oil is used is very important to remember, because some, if applied or taken in excess, or if too strong, have the reverse effect to that which is desired. For example, a low concentration of peppermint oil applied to an itchy skin will relieve the irritation; a strong concentration will aggravate the condition.

Similarly, *digitalis*, which is from the essential oil of foxglove, is poisonous in high concentrations, but used carefully in medicine, it is very effective in relieving heart conditions.

It can be seen therefore that, when mixing oils for use in aromatherapy as well as in medicine, it is very important to use the correct concentration of essential oil, and also to realize that with many oils it does not necessarily follow that the more we use the better will be the result!

The high rate of evaporation of essential oils was mentioned earlier, and this is sometimes considered when mixing a well-balanced product. This volatility rate varies in different oils, and most essences fall into one of the following three classifi-cations:

**top notes**       —   the quickest to evaporate,
                        the most stimulating and uplifting to
                        mind and body.

**middle notes** —   moderately volatile,
                        primarily affect the functions of the
                        body e.g., digestion, menstruation and
                        the general metabolism of the body.

**base notes**      —   slower to evaporate (if mixed with top
                        note oil, it can help to 'hold back' the
                        volatility of that oil. The most sedating
                        and relaxing.

## HOW ESSENTIAL OILS ARE OBTAINED

Before distillation was invented, aromatic oils and waves were extracted from the plants by hand expression, enfleurage and maceration.

**Expression** is confined to the citrus family, and the rinds used to be literally squeezed by hand until the oil glands or globules burst. The oil was collected in a sponge, which was squeezed into a container when saturated. This method is still used, but by machines instead of hands. Expressed oils can be classed as essential oils.

**Enfleurage** was the method used for extracting the aroma from flowers, by placing the chosen flower heads on a glass bed covered with purified fat. The aromatic constituents were absorbed by the fat, the flowers removed, a new covering of flower heads put on and so on, repeating the process until the fat was saturated with the aroma and any other plant compo-nents soluble in fat. The resultant compound was called a 'pomade' and was often used in this state as an ointment or perfume. Enfleurage is still used as a method of extraction, but is usually carried to its second stage, which is to dissolve the pomade in alcohol. Fat is insoluble in alcohol but the aromatic molecules readily dissolve in it. The resultant liquid is then carefully heated, and as the alcohol evaporates first, the aromatic liquid is left in the container. Oils obtained by enfleurage are not classed as essential oils, and if taken to the liquid stage, are known as absolutes.

**Maceration** is similar to enfleurage and is a method by which one can make an aromatic oil at home in a ready diluted state. The flowers or leaves are crushed to rupture some of the oil glands or cells, then put into warm vegetable oil and put in a warm place. The vegetable oil absorbs the aromatic molecules and the flowers are strained off. A fresh lot of flowers or leaves is put into the re-warmed 'carrier' base, and this process is repeated until the vegetable oil is concentrated enough; the resultant liquid can be used as it is for massage self-application or in the making of home-made herbal creams.

**Solvent extraction** is a method used to produce aromatic concretes and oils for the food and perfume industries. It is a very complicated process, using a volatile solvent in a closed apparatus and a vacuum still, which yields a solid consisting of the aromatic constituents and other plant extracts, including the natural waxes and colour. This substance is called a 'concrete', which is then mixed with alcohol (later evaporated off) to remove the waxes, leaving an absolute, normally thicker liquid than an oil obtained by distillation. These absolutes are, of course, very expensive and usually have a heavier, sweeter aroma than essential oils. The purity of the oil is dependent on how well the solvent is evaporated off. Absolutes always contain a residue of the solvents used in this complicated process of extraction and are also easily (and often) adulterated by the addition of synthetic chemicals, therefore great care should be exercised when buying these oils – their litre price can vary in some instances by £1,000 or more, depending on the quality. Absolutes and resins are not classed as essential oils and are never prescribed for internal use.

**Steam distillation is** the only method which produces an essential oil. Primitive methods were used prior to the arrival of Avicenna, an eleventh century Arabian physician, who greatly improved the process of distillation as a method of extracting essential oils from plants. Arnaldo de Vilanova (a Spaniard) probably gave the first authentic written description of the process of distillation in the thirteenth century, and may even have introduced this art to Europe.

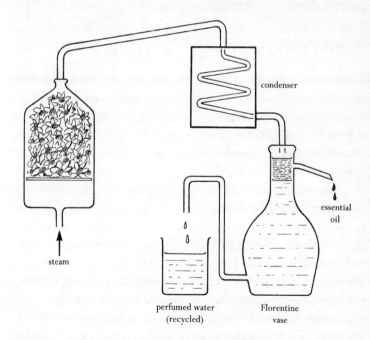

*Figure 1*. Steam distillation.

Figure 1 (which may remind us of school days in the lab!) shows clearly how steam distillation is carried out. It depends on the density of the oil extracted as to whether it will float above the water, or sink below it, after condensation. This method makes use of the high volatility rate of essential oils plus the fact that they are mainly insoluble in water. However, some components *are* water soluble – and when plants such as rose or melissa are distilled, the same water is used over and over again throughout the distillation process (called cohobation) and eventually becomes saturated with these components. The result is a better essential oil, because molecules are not lost to fresh water each time new plant material is put into the still. The resulting floral water is more concentrated than usual and is diluted before use.

## THE PURITY OF ESSENTIAL OILS

From the account of the methods of extraction, the substances in which essential oils dissolve will be apparent. Mainly, they do not dissolve in water; they readily dissolve in alcohol; they dissolve in oil (vegetable or mineral) and they dissolve in fat. This information can help us to recognize a poor quality essential oil.

All essential oils are relatively expensive, though prices cover a wide range (depending mainly on percentage yield). If we see a low percentage yield, e.g., rose or jasmine, at a fairly low/medium price, it is probably not even a lower quality pure oil, but adulterated in some way, perhaps diluted in a solvent of some sort, or with added synthetic oils, the perfume of which can be a very good imitation of the real thing. So beware!

It is also difficult to compare prices of authentic essential oils, because one firm may import Chinese geranium, which is a much lower price than Bourbon geranium. Mysore sandalwood

(East Indian and by far the best therapeutically) is at least twice the price of Australian sandalwood, and so on.

As with most things the price is comparable with the quality, and the quality is definitely comparable with the results when essential oils are used for therapeutic purposes.

Synthetic substitutes are generally quite successful for cookery and perfumery, but it cannot be stressed enough that for the purpose of aromatherapy **only the best and purest** essential oils will give the desired effect.

By the way – essential oils are *not* greasy, though the name certainly suggests this. Most of them do not leave an oily mark on blotting paper (as would a drop of other oils we know, like corn oil) and their power of penetration through the skin and adjacent tissue is very great.

## STORAGE OF ESSENTIAL OILS

Oils, as we already know, have a high evaporation rate; they are also sensitive to light, and care should be taken when using and storing them. Always replace the bottle top each time it is used.

- because of their volatility they must be kept in tightly stoppered bottles
- because they are sensitive to light, which can destroy them, they must be kept in dark bottles
- because polythene tends to absorb essential oils they must be kept in glass or metal containers

In short, essential oils should be kept in air-tight, dark glass in a cool dark place for maximum shelf life.

For best results do not store ready mixed in a carrier oil for any length of time (maximum eighteen months). Essential oils in their pure state have a much longer life – several years if stored correctly.

*chapter three*

# THE SKIN

The skin is the largest organ we have, covering and protecting the whole body, and it deserves to be taken care of. Any other organ which may be out of order and causing us discomfort is given immediate attention. But often the skin does not cause much discomfort when dry or cracked, or over oily, so we tend to think we are doing our best with it if we keep off soap and use skin care products for the prevailing condition.

In fact, a healthy skin reflects a healthy body and a blemished, flaking or irritable skin is often the result of some other part being out of order. We all know how our hair looks and feels when we are in low health; sometimes just a simple cold can make it lank and out of condition (even though it is dead matter according to science!)

Owners of spotty or blemished skins often forget that what is *eaten* affects the skin (and hair) and if greasy or convenience foods form a large part of their diet, the the skin reflects this in its lack of glow, and perhaps spots or blackheads show themselves.

Stress can also affect the skin, causing it to be patchy and sensitive to certain products. Here it is necessary to get at the root cause, the stress or anxiety, and treat this in order to improve the skin.

Imperfect skin can also be due to hereditary causes. For instance, if you, or a relation, have, or have had, eczema, asthma or hay fever, it is possible for you to have blemished skin, with dry patches. It is likely that you would presume yourself to be allergic to certain soaps or cosmetics, when in reality it is the eczema connection showing on your skin.

Similarly, if you suffer from psoriasis, you may think you are stuck with it except when you are using a cream from the doctor. Nothing completely cures psoriasis, except perhaps continual exposure to sunshine – difficult in England! – but solariums and sunbeds, if taken fairly regularly, can often keep psoriasis down to a minimum.

People who have dermatitis are often given a steroid cream to clear it. It does clear it, quickly, but there are side effects if the cream is used too often or for too long.

Quite a number of people, usually female, suffer from a super sensitive skin and find it very difficult to discover a brand of skin care which will not bring up an allergic reaction. Very often these ladies use a simple soap to avoid reactions, but of course, although it does the cleaning job well, it doesn't moisturize or feed or care for the skin in a way which will improve it.

Another sad story!

However, essential oils can help all these cases (see Case Histories. Chap. 13.) and many more besides (including headaches and sinus problems!), by the use of good skin care products containing essential oils for their particular condition. And so, by spending *no extra time* on the daily skin care routine, many facial and skin problems can be dealt with automatically.

There is a range of skin care products which I have designed myself, mainly for the person who has a special problem with his or her skin. There are cleansers, toners, moisturizers, night cream, hand lotion, body lotion and masks – all designed to treat as well as take care of the skin. (see Useful Addresses). All creams and lotions are hypo-allergenic and are based on pure plant extracts. There is no lanolin in any of them, as lanolin (from sheep's wool) is responsible for a lot of allergies. There is no mineral oil in the moisturizers and night cream so maximum penetration is effected, to take care of the growing cells below the surface of the top skin. There is no animal product used and no perfume added. These two are other ingredients which can often be responsible for many allergic reactions.

So before we even start mentioning essential oils, the products are suitable for a very sensitive skin, which is important in itself.

Then we come to the interesting part. To the basic product different essential oils are added to help different types of skin; not just sensitive, dry, combination and oily, but eczema, dermatitis, sinus blockage, psoriasis, broken veins, stress, insomnia, persistent headaches, etc. By using these every day you can help to clear up your problem, yet do nothing more than carry out normal skin care routine! And in most cases it costs no more than many well-known brands.

For those who are not accustomed to using a skin care routine I am going to set out a programme for you to follow. Those of you who do not like cleansing creams or lotions because you like to rinse your face with water will be very pleased to know that cleansers are now available, including my own, which are water soluble and can be rinsed off in the same way as soap if wished.

## *THE SKIN*

The surface of our skin (the epidermis) is completely made up of dead, yes, dead, skin cells. In a baby and young child these are continuously and quickly thrown off by the newer cells underneath, which in their turn are thrown off themselves. A child's skin is normally moist, rounded and smooth because of the speedy regeneration of new cells everywhere in the body, and equally speedy throwing off of dead ones. As we get older, of course, the regeneration of new cells slows down (not just in the skin) and old dead cells are slower in being thrown off. This can be responsible, in part, for dry skin, and is certainly an aid in the acquiring of wrinkles, where the dead cells collect in the little furrows of the skin and our facial expressions push them into line formation.

Soap, although a fairly efficient cleanser, usually has an alkaline base, and for the elasticity of the skin to be preserved, alkaline substances are not good. This is because the skin is slightly acid (in order to kill bacteria which may invade the tissue) and using an alkaline cleanser removes this needed acidity. It is also very drying, hence oily skinned people think soap is good for them. Certainly oily skinned people stay younger-looking for longer, but often they pay for the privilege by having a spotty or open-pored skin in their late teens (due mainly to hormonal changes and also to incorrect diet).

Underneath the epidermis we have a layer of skin called the dermis. This is alive, and contains all the blood vessels, nerve endings, oil and sweat glands. Here, new skin cells are made and pushed upwards, and as they reach the epidermis they flatten, die off and are eventually thrown off the skin surface.

The skin is waterproof and only the epidermis gets wet and needs to be dried off. Because of this quality, not many substances can penetrate the skin – in fact many doctors pooh-pooh skin creams as nothing but surface protectors. With lotions containing mineral oil we know this to be true – they give the effect of moisturizing the skin because they *do* keep the *surface* moist. But we will learn in a later chapter that mineral oil does not penetrate the skin too well, therefore no improvement can be given to the living cells underneath the top skin – we are just keeping the top skin temporarily moist. (See Case Histories (Mrs F) on p. 198.)

Creams containing lanolin are similar in their non-effectiveness as skin regenerators. Lanolin particles are usually too large to penetrate the skin, as anyone who uses night cream rich in lanolin will know – not only does the face look greasy, but the cream penetrates the pillow more than the face. Vegetable oil based creams and lotions, on the other hand, are able to have slight penetration into the skin

Essential oils, as we have seen, are *highly* penetrative and can reach the small blood capillaries in the dermis, from whence they are carried in the blood to do something useful. At the same time, if the *right* oils are added, the skin can be rejuvenated, i.e., better quality skin cells are made, because they are fed with the right ingredients; so they look smoother and feel softer and less dry or less oily (as the case may be) as they reach the skin surface and die off.

Opening onto the skin are two special types of gland: the sweat gland and the sebaceous or oil glands. The latter produce a natural oil called sebum, which comes onto the skin surface via the hair follicle. So where there are no hairs at all, there is no oil, i.e., palms of hands, soles of feet, eye area.

The job of sebum is to lubricate the skin and preserve its elasticity.

The sweat glands produce a watery, yet slightly oily, liquid we call perspiration, which escapes onto the skin surface via pore openings. The palms of the hands have the most sweat glands, though there are many present in the soles of the feet, the armpits and on the forehead and nose too.

Sweat glands eliminate body waste and toxins and also provide the body's own cooling system, so when we are hot, through exerting ourselves, these glands send out extra moisture to help cool the body down. Normally, to maintain body temperature, we don't notice our sweat glands working but in wind, sun and central heating especially, this normal amount of moisture produced evaporates too quickly, leaving the skin drier than it should be. This is why it is essential to use a moisturizer daily to help to counteract this loss, especially on skiing or sun-seeking holidays.

The sweat glands work *together* to keep the surface of the skin supple and balanced. If one type of gland is over-or under-productive, then this shows itself in an oily or dry skin type. Using the correct moisturizer for the skin type helps to balance this and keep the skin supple. Even people with over-productive oil glands need a moisturizer to replace the *moisture* lost, which is causing the oil to predominate. *But* it must then be a moisturizer which contains a minimal amount of oil, and is mainly water in a light emulsion.

Every time the face and neck are washed, a moisturizer should be applied, because all the natural oil and moisture on the skin surface has been washed off; thus to protect the skin a moisture lotion or moisture cream should be used on the face and neck afterwards.

This does three things for us:

- counteracts unnatural moisture loss.
- keeps oil and moisture content of skin balanced.
- protects pore openings from dirt and make-up, which can clog them and cause blackheads and spots.

You can see now that everyone needs a moisturizer (even men should use one!) but not everyone needs a night cream. A night cream lubricates the skin and (provided a good veg-etable based one is used) also feeds the growing cells in the dermis, ensuring improvement in elasticity. Oily skinned people do not generally need a night cream until they feel their skin is beginning to dry out on the cheek area, then one should be used around the eyes, (never use a lanolin based cream around the eyes), on the cheeks and all over the neck area. Remember, there are not any oil glands on the eyes and very few on the neck, so don't neglect the areas that need feeding just because you have a very oily strip down the centre of your face.

A night cream does two important things:

- replaces oil where glands are not functioning properly, or are slowing down due to getting older.
- keeps skin well lubricated and so minimizes the risk of early wrinkles due to loss of skin elasticity.

Two other areas which need feeding as we get older, because the pores are not producing so much moisture, are our hands and feet. Use of a body lotion after each shower or bath can take care of dry feet, legs and hands, and hand lotion, applied every time the hands are washed, helps to keep them supple and moist, and there is one on the market which is also particularly good for chapped hands. (See Useful Addresses).

Special areas need treatment with masks:

- very oily skin down centre of face.
- very dry skin on face and neck.
- fine wrinkle lines at side of eyes and mouth, forehead and upper lip.
- sallow skin, lacking tone and colour.
- dry backs of heels, elbows and knees and dry hands.

Dry and sallow areas need a feeding mask or a mask which will activate the blood circulation, thus bringing nutrients to the area. Very oily areas need a mask which will clean out pores and oil glands.

Wrinkle lines need a mask to clean out dead skin cells from furrows (use a moisturizer immediately afterwards).

Sensitive skins do not often need a treatment mask, but natural yogurt with liquidized cucumber will soothe and freshen any type of skin, including a sensitive one.

## SKIN CARE ROUTINE

The aim of skin care is to encourage all types of skin to become normal through the correct use of well chosen skin care products, and combination skins should use (over the whole face and neck) the cleanser and moisturizer to suit the area which is the greatest problem. Those with oily panels should use a mask to rectify these, and a cleanser and moisturizer (over the whole face and neck) to suit the cheek area.

Caring for the skin takes no longer than washing with soap and water. The only additional few seconds is the use of a toner and moisturizer.

Every night:
Cleanse face and neck thoroughly – rinse off.
Apply toner on cotton wool.
Put night cream (or moisturizer when you don't need night cream) on face, neck and eyes *(or moisture lotion if very oily).
Eye creams and gels without lanolin or mineral oil can be used on any skin type.
* Not on eyes if cream is lanolin based.
Every morning:
Wipe face, neck and eyes with toner on cotton wool.
(Not necessary to cleanse again unless you want to).

Apply moisturizer to face, neck and eyes* then make-up if worn.

* Not on eyes if cream is lanolin based.

If at any time after this you want to wear make-up you need to re-moisturize immediately before applying it, or cleanse, tone and moisturize first if more than four hours later.

Once a week (twice for an oily panel) a treatment mask should be used if it is needed. People with a normal skin need only use a mask every now and again, except for the yogurt and cucumber type, which can be used as often as you wish.

It is very important that you use a spatula with jars of cream. Not only is it economical, but also it prevents your putting in any bacteria which may be under your nails and may multiply in the cream.

The following table should be of help, and if you have a combination skin use the cleanser and moisturizer to suit the cheek area, and use a mask for open pores and blackheads on the oily panel once or twice a week.

| | Sensitive | Oily | Normal | Dry |
|---|---|---|---|---|
| Cleansing Cream | ● | | ● | ● |
| Cleansing Milk | ● | ● | ● | |
| Alcohol-free Toning Lotion | ● | ● | ● | ● |
| Moisture Lotion (lanolin & mineral oil-free) | ● | ● | ● | |
| Moisture Cream (lanolin & mineral oil-free) | ● | | ● | ● |
| Night Cream (lanolin & mineral oil-free) | ● | ● | ● | ● |
| Eye Cream & Gels (lanolin & mineral oil-free) | ● | ● | ● | ● |
| Mask for open pores and blackheads | | ● | ● | ● |
| Feeding Mask | ● | ● | ● | ● |
| Mask for stimulating the blood circulation | | ● | ● | ● |
| Yogurt and Cucumber | ● | ● | ● | ● |

## BASIC SKIN CARE PROCEDURE

## Cleansing

| PRODUCT | METHOD | ACTION |
|---|---|---|
| **Cleansing Creams**<br>(use a spatula)<br>Effectively cleanses normal or dry skin. Very dry skins should always use a cream. | 1. Small amount on finger tips; place fingers of both hands together.<br><br>2. Using both hands massage cream in upward and outward circles over neck and face.<br><br>3. Eye circles should start on upper lid at nose and come to temple, returning to nose underneath the eye (One continuous circle).<br><br>4. Rinse off with water, or wipe off with damp cotton wool. | 1. Removes stale make-up from skin surface.<br><br>2. Removes accumulated skin secretions.<br><br>3. Removes dust and dirt.<br>(Excellent for removing make-up round the eyes for any skin-type.)<br><br>4. Helps to normalize a dry skin. |
| **Cleansing Milks**<br>These have the same properties as cleansing creams, but in the form of a lotion, which is suitable for any skin which is not very dry. | As for cleansing creams. | 1. Removes stale make-up from skin surface.<br><br>2. Removes accumulated skin secretions.<br><br>3. Removes dust and dirt.<br><br>4. Helps to normalize an oily skin. |

## PRODUCT

**Alcohol-free Toning Lotions**

A natural toner to freshen, tone and re-vitalise the skin. Suitable for all skin types, even the most sensitive, as it is non-drying.

### METHOD

1. Moisten cotton wool with toner (hold on bottle and tip up twice for correct amount).
2. Wipe gently over face and neck, upwards and outwards.

### ACTION

1. Refreshes and cools skin.
2. Tones facial muscles.
3. Removes any remaining traces of cleanser plus make-up or dirt.
4. Can be used as a cleanser where make-up has not been worn. i.e., first thing in the morning.

## Conditioning

## PRODUCT

**Masks** for open pores & blackheads (use a spatula).

### METHOD

1. Small amount on back of hand.
2. Massage into the skin in small circles for 2 to 3 minutes, wherever the problem is, keeping it moist. (Dip finger in water if necessary.)
3. Do not use *under* eyes but on corners of eyes and along upper lip to help prevent premature wrinkling.
4. Rinse off with warm water and pat dry.
5. Follow with moisture lotion or cream.

### ACTION

1. Normalizes an oily skin.
2. Stimulates and refreshes.
3. Gentle abrasive action lifts out dead skin cells lying in valleys of skin, thus making wrinkle-lines less obvious.
4. Helps remove blackheads.
5. Helps spots (unless medical in origin).
6. Refines open pores.
7. Deep cleanses a greasy skin.
8. Smooths rough skin (heels, elbows, etc.)

| PRODUCT | METHOD | ACTION |
|---|---|---|
| **Feeding Masks**<br>(use a spatula)<br>Mixed with equal part of natural yogurt makes a superb soothing and cooling mask. | 1. Take about a teaspoonful and spread *quickly* and evenly over the skin of face and neck (even under the eyes). Do not rub in.<br>2. Leave for the time stated.<br>3. Rinse off with warm water and pat dry.<br>4. Follow with moisture lotion or cream. | 1. Normalizes a dry skin.<br>2. Refreshes and smooths.<br>3. Gently stimulates circulation.<br>4. Softens dead skin cells on surface which are removed with mask.<br>5. Refines pores.<br>6. Smooths and softens hands. |
| **Masks** to promote blood circulation<br>(use a spatula)<br>Effective treatment mask for skin improvement but must be used with care. Can be mixed with natural yogurt on a sensitive skin. | 1. As in 1 above – Feeding Masks.<br>2. Sensitive skin – leave for *1 minute only* on first treatment, increasing to 3 minutes after 4 to 5 treatments. Sallow, dull skin – leave for 15 to 20 minutes. (Adjust or skin types in between).<br>3. and 4. as above. | 1. Normalizes a sensitive skin.<br>2. Activates blood circulation to promote healthy skin.<br>3. Acts as mild skin peeling, removing dead skin cells from surface.<br>4. Refines pores.<br>5. Good feeding mask for hands and feet. |

*Note:* Always remove *any* mask immediately if prickling sensation occurs before the required time.

## Protecting

| PRODUCT | METHOD | ACTION |
|---|---|---|
| **Moisture Lotions** (without lanolin or mineral oil)<br><br>A light lotion to give an oily or normal skin the right amount of moisture needed to keep the skin supple. Non-greasy, therefore excellent for keeping eyelids well moistened and supple. | 1. Small amount on tips of fingers; place fingers of both hands together.<br>2. 'Run' over face *and neck* with tips of fingers.<br>3. Blend lotion into face and neck with outward and upward movements.<br>4. Do not forget to include the eyelids! These *need* moisture protection. | 1. Helps to normalize an oily skin.<br>2. Keeps skin's natural moisture balance correct, by replacing moisture lost through sweat glands.<br>3. Forms a barrier to help prevent dust, dirt and make-up going into pores. |
| **Moisture Creams** (without lanolin or mineral oil) (use a spatula)<br><br>A day cream to give a normal to dry skin the right amount of moisture to keep the skin supple and free from flaking. | As in Moisture Lotions.<br>Do not forget eyes and neck. | 1. Helps to normalize a dry skin.<br>2. and 3. as in Moisture Lotions.<br>4. Helps to maintain a higher level of moisture in the skin. |

## Preserving

| PRODUCT | METHOD | ACTION |
|---|---|---|
| **Night Creams** (without lanolin) (use a spatula) Specially formulated to keep a high degree of moisture in the skin and aid in the retardation of ageing. Suitable for all skin types, because they should be completely non-greasy. | As in Moisture Lotions and do not forget eyes and neck. *Note:* Oily skins should use once a week. Dry skins should use every night. | 1. Softens and beautifies skin. 2. Keeps wrinkles at bay. 3. Helps to preserve natural elasticity of skin. |
| **Eye Creams and Gels** (without lanolin) (use a spatula) Specially made for the extra sensitive skin around the eyes, they will help to prevent wrinkles and keep skin supple. | 1. Take a very small amount onto ring fingers only. 2. Circle round eyes from nose to temple on upper lid and back to nose under eye. Continue circling. 3. Can also be used above upper lip where fine vertical lines start to form. | 1. Keeps skin around eyes soft and supple. 2. Softens existing lines. 3. Helps prevent new lines forming. |

# chapter four

# COMPLEMENTARY THERAPIES AND HOLISM

There are over a hundred different therapies which come under the heading of alternative and complementary therapies and it is important to understand that each therapy is a discipline in its own right and should not be confused or linked in the mind with any other therapy. The basic principle of any current complementary therapy should be holistic, which means that the whole person should be treated — not just the symptoms, as so often happens in allopathic medicine. Naturally, this depends on the attitude of mind of the practitioner, rather than the individual discipline itself, and a caring therapist of any discipline will have this approach, looking at the complete lifestyle of the person needing help; the kind of food eaten, the amount, if any, of exercise taken, the environment in which the person lives, the occupation or type of employment, relationships with family and leisure pursuits (again, if any) and very importantly, attitude and outlook on life in general.

All these, added up, make the whole person. We already are familiar with the sayings 'we are what we eat' and 'we are what we think' — they have been proved over and over again to be true. If we eat correctly, think only positive thoughts and manage to avoid severe stress, we could stay healthy without needing much help from either orthodox or complementary medicine – except of course, in emergencies. Life in the latter half of the 20th century has accelerated in pace. Stress, once a word which hardly existed, is now designated a medical illness; its incidence is growing at such an alarming rate that it could be one of the main causes of illness before the first decade of the 21st century has ended.

There are disciplines of which the principle aim is to reduce stress (stress therapy) and those which specialize in helping people by influencing the way they think (positive thinking and mind dynamics); there are those which specialize in advice on diets (nutrition) and those which specialize in relaxation techniques (yoga, meditation, hypnosis). Holistic therapists qualified in complementary disciplines will look at all these aspects when assessing the whole person; they will normally have gained sufficient knowledge on nutrition, positive thinking and exercise during the study of their own discipline to be able to recommend an improvement in lifestyle as a basis for correcting the health problem being suffered. If they feel a client needs extra help from one of the above or to any other therapy in which they are not qualified, they will refer them on, should they feel it is in their client's best interests.

Some complementary therapies are more popular (and possibly more efficacious) than others and there is only space here to mention a few of the most popular. Aromatherapy is one of these and is being practised not only by individual therapists but also in many hospitals: to help problems which are a result of side effects from allopathic drugs; to relax people in intensive care by reducing the heart rate and slowing the breathing and to ease the suffering of those in palliative care. It is also used extensively in midwifery; during pregnancy – to help problems like backache and swollen ankles and prevent stretch marks; three weeks before, and during, labour;

to ease labour pains and stimulate the uterus to contract; after the birth – to help heal bruised or torn perineums; help correct feeding problems and often to boost the immune system in those suffering from postnatal depression.

## ENERGY BASED THERAPIES

Not everyone is at ease with therapies which are based on energy flow (e.g. the meridian lines used in acupuncture and shiatsu and the reflex points in reflexology) as they cannot be proved to exist by X-ray (as can the accepted systems of the body). Such people need to remember that electricity and television are fantasic proof of energy existing without being able to see it. Kirlian photography is believed to show the energy field around the body, which shows a different result when the body is in a healthy state from when the body is in a state of illness – and before and after beneficial treatment.

Einstein proved that energy and matter are two forms of the same universal substance, therefore we are all composed of – energy. We are familiar with energies in nature like wind and heat; energy in nature also takes the form of flowers and trees. Our energy takes the form of a human body and has tangible and intangible forces, the latter of which we take for granted, for example, speech and thought – particularly thought. This last is our innermost, secret being and it cannot be seen, touched or X-rayed – at the moment!

The whole concept of the universe, life and energy is so awe-inspiring that one has to believe that there is a Force, in control of it all. For me, this force is God, who has been responsible for so many amazing and positive things in my life. To some people, this force is Universal Energy, but whatever name you give to this undeniable and wondrous power, whether you believe in God, or simply Universal Energy, it is in reality one and the same Being. 'God created everything in heaven and on earth, the seen and the unseen things, including spiritual powers ...' (Colossians 1.16). There is otherwise, no rational explanation.

All complementary therapies work on the principle of keeping the body's energy at a level conducive to good health and there are therapies which actually use energy (such as the meridian lines mentioned above). Whatever complementary therapy you choose, the mind is such that what you believe will help you will generally do so.

In our Western medical books nine bodily systems are known: circulatory, digestive, excretory, glandular, muscular, nervous, reproductive, respiratory and skeletal. Each of these can be located physically – and seen; the mechanisms and the way in which they function can be logically worked out and demonstrated. Any disorder in a system has always been treated in Western medicine by addressing the symptoms produced by the disorder, without regard to the underlying cause, although, no doubt because of the growth and success of complementary therapies, some orthodox practitioners now place greater emphasis on the importance of cause and effect in health.

The Western world in general has just begun to accept (and this acceptance is steadily growing) that less easily explained 'systems' do exist in the human body, systems which, in the East, have been used for hundreds of years to diagnose and to treat the nine systems we know – and their related organs. The 'meridian lines system' in acupuncture and acupressure is one example and the 'zones system' in press point therapy or reflexology is another (both are related to energy flow in the body). This is not to say that one of these approaches (Eastern and Western) is better than the other, but that both can be used, one to complement the other, in order to provide a more complete healing system: we need them both.

## Each To His Own

Most people know that homoeopathy is a discipline in its own right and do not confuse it in their minds with any other complementary therapy. It is the same with reflexology, kinesiology, Chinese medicine, etc. Unfortunately, this is not so with aromatherapy, as people often believe this *includes* shiatsu, healing with crystals and other energy type therapies. In fact, many aromatherapy schools teach the principles of yin and yang and the use of crystals as *part* of their aromatherapy course, which may be responsible for the misunderstanding. As each of these are separate disciplines – although they may be used individually or together in one treatment – they should be taught separately, giving the full time required to each one if a qualification is to be awarded. People are individuals and often a discipline which suits one doesn't necessarily suit another. Also, using more than one therapy – as a combined treatment – may be more efficacious on certain problems and certain people. This is why a complementary therapist usually has a qualification in more than one discipline.

Because of these possible misunderstandings, a therapist who is using more than one therapy or technique should inform the client of the type of therapy or therapies being offered in a treatment. They should not be offering something like crystal, colour or aura healing as though it were *part* of an aromatherapy treatment; successful treatments in these other disciplines can be carried out by those qualified in them, but the client should be informed at the outset that more than one therapy is to be used – just to make sure the client too realizes that the therapies are separate.

## *AROMATHERAPY INDEPENDENCE*

Naturally, my passion and interest lies in making sure that aromatherapy in particular is recognized as a therapy which uses only essential oils (and the hands, of course!) – and that as such, it is a unique therapy able to stand alone or be used in conjunction with other equally independent therapies.

Although, fortunately, most churches recognize that aromatherapy is only to do with essential oils, I have had extensive correspondence with some church leaders who believe it to be part and parcel with Eastern therapies, such as those mentioned above – plus others of similar nature, which they see as 'supernatural' – and in some cases, even 'wicked'! I am sure the problem is mainly their fear of the unknown or 'unprovable', but it also springs out of the New Age era, when complementary therapies were just emerging and Universal Energy was the new explanation for those who were unsure of their belief in God to explain the wonders of existence. However, the healing which is attributed to Jesus in the Bible could not be explained or 'proved' by science – it was literally God's energy at work!

I always explain to these church people that no other therapy (complementary or so-called New Age) should be linked with aromatherapy (aromatherapy and herbal medicine can be classed together under the heading of phytotherapy – i.e. plant medicine in general), and that as aromatherapists use only extracts from plants which were put into this world by the very Creator on whom they (and myself, as it happens) base their beliefs, they should be very happy about it! After all, most drugs used in modern medicine are man-made – although even here plants were the starting point for the synthesis of drugs – and all healing plants are made by the God in whom they believe implicitly!

The strict meaning of aromatherapy is 'the use of essential oils to maintain or improve the general well-being of the whole person' – body, mind and spirit – and they are able to do this on their own, without help from shiatsu, crystals, reflexology – or even massage. Essential oils are used nowadays in hospitals – rarely with full body massage (although often with massage of the hands or feet); they are used in compresses, inhalations and baths – and it is important that the discipline is recognized for what it is – an effective therapy – independent, without being linked with other therapies; this is not to say that other therapies are not effective – many are, but in *their* own right also!

Aromatherapy was originally taught in the UK with full body massage. This has given the wrong picture, as massage also is an independent discipline, and there are many other ways of using essential oils successfully apart from a complete massage, in order to improve our health. In France, where the word aromatherapy originated, massage is not even one of the methods by which naturothérapeutes and some doctors (who have also qualified in phytotherapy) use essential oils, although they do, when appropriate, apply them to specific parts of the body, e.g. the chest, in cases of bronchitis. The main method of use in France is by ingestion (against infection), in place of antibiotics, which can themselves cause further health problems due to unwanted secondary effects – and also the body can become immune to their action.

There are some disciplines whose principles help complementary therapists not qualified in that particular discipline to carry out their holistic assessment, for example, reflex testing on the feet and kinesiology testing, both of which can be used as diagnostic tools after a preliminary course (full training is required in both of these to use them in giving a treatment). Another diagnostic tool sometimes used is iridology, but again, this cannot be used as a treatment without full training.

Although separate therapies, shiatsu and reflexology were the two therapies first to be confused with – and sometimes taught with – aromatherapy. Therefore, to illustrate how completely different they are, I have given a brief overview of these two disciplines.

## Finding a Good Aromatherapist

In 1997, HRH the Prince of Wales suggested that a steering committee should be set up to consider the current relationship between orthodox, complementary and alternative medicine in the UK. The ensuing report calls for common training standards in the various disciplines, which, in my opinion, is not before time. There are some basic skills necessary to all complementary therapists and there are skills applicable to each individual therapy, though the variation in training standards of each is quite considerable in many cases, as each therapy has a number of professional bodies to which therapists can belong – if indeed they are qualified enough to join one of these. It would be a great help, both to therapists and to the public, if each therapy had but one (or at worst, two) professional bodies, as standards would have to be at the highest level known for that particular therapy.

There are too many aromatherapy associations unfortunately, but there are moves afoot at the moment to persuade them all to come together as one body, which will benefit not only therapists (who will then have only one subscription to pay) but also the public (who would have an idea of the type and standard of treatment to expect from a therapist member).

Until this becomes a reality, always ask if the therapist you want to see belongs to one of the associations who set a professional standard, e.g. International Society of Professional

Aromatherapists (ISPA), Institute of Aromatic Medicine (IAM), International Federation of Aromatherapists (IFA), Register of Qualified Aromatherapists (RQA): this way you will be sure of a holistic and complete treatment. Ask also if the therapist specializes in, or uses, any other complementary therapy, as this will give you an idea of what to expect. All therapists belonging to the above associations will select essential oils for your individual problems, having first looked at you holistically and offered advice where (or if) needed on lifestyle and nutritionary needs. If you go to someone who is not a member of one of these associations, you may be given a massage (usually that is good) with oils that have been pre-mixed to suit a variety of conditions – and you will be given the one which is nearest to your symptoms. You have been warned!

## SHIATSU

Let's start with shiatsu (finger pressure). This is a massage originating from the East and is sometimes referred to as acupuncture without needles or 'acupressure'. It is based on energy flow and to understand it more easily it is necessary to look at the principles of yin and yang.

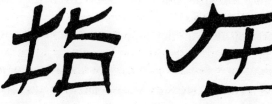

**SHI** **ATSU**

*Figure 2*. Shiatsu.

In the East, all natural forces (or energies) are divided into two categories; passive (or negative) forces and active (or positive) forces, called yin and yang respectively. Examples of other yin/yang characteristics are: weak/strong, empty/full, dark/light. These forces complement and also balance each other, both in nature and in the human body. Even if we don't understand (or believe in) yin and yang, we can see how the idea originated, as nature (and humans) balances their energies in a similar way. For example:

- sunshine usually follows rain and rain follows sunshine
- wind or storms are usually followed by calm and *vice versa*
- day follows night; night follows day (always!)
- sleep and daytime pursuits of humans alternate to keep the body in balance
- the human mind has alternating moods of low and high spirits

In the human body there are invisible lines called meridians, along which the body energy is said to flow and along which are points (called tsubos) connected with all the systems in our body, both physical and mental. These complement one another and are called either yin or yang meridians:

- yang meridians flow down the body (from fingertips to shoulders in the arms)
- yin meridians flow up the body (from shoulders to fingertips in the arms)

No person is completely yang or completely yin, but an ever-changing balance of the two; nevertheless, essentially, a person follows either a yin-type or yang-type pattern of behaviour.

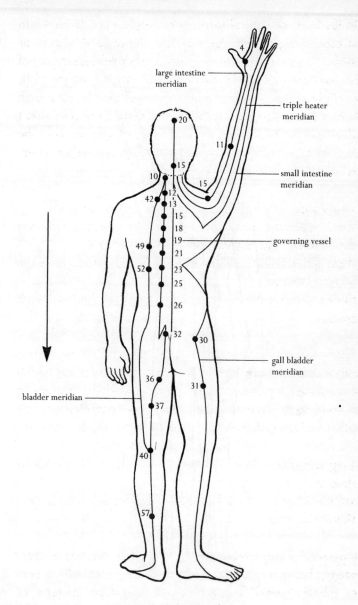

*Figure 3.* Yang Meridians.

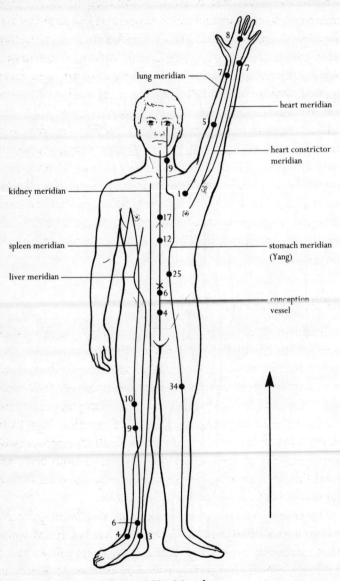

*Figure 4.* Yin Meridians.

Shiatsu pressure points are quite difficult to find without training in the subject and much experience is needed to keep the body in good general health – and/or relieve symptoms which show themselves – using this therapy. Treatment is based on accuracy in direction and type of pressure being applied to these points, following the meridian flow on a person who is basically yin (slow, gentle pressure and slow release) and moving against the meridian flow (quick, strong pressure and quick release) on someone who has a mainly yang character. All this sounds very confusing – indeed it *is* confusing – and one really needs to visit an experienced shiatsu therapist to benefit fully from this type of massage. Although there is no specific shiatsu in a pure aromatherapy treatment, many of these pressure points are automatically covered during massage.

## REFLEXOLOGY

Reflexology is also known as 'zone therapy', 'compression massage' and 'press point therapy' and many books have been written on the subject. Some aromatherapists use the reflexes as a diagnostic tool before doing an aromatherapy treatment, as it is a speedy and accurate method of client assessment; this is not, and should not be thought to be, a reflexology treatment. A full reflexology treatment can be both a preventative and treatment of disease, and can also relax both body and mind (like an aromatherapy treatment) from the world's most popular 'disease' at the present time – stress.

The nearest we can get to a definition of reflexology is that it is an ancient Eastern technique which makes use of somewhat mysterious connecting pathways or energy flow lines in the body, which connect from bodily systems to points on the feet (and hands, ears and tongue). These lines are as complicated as our nervous system, but very different. In order for you to understand the difference between the reflexes in reflexology and the reflexes connected to the nervous system, the latter is briefly explained below.

## Our Nervous System

The job of the nervous system is to convey information from the world outside and conditions inside our body to the brain, and also to transmit instructions from the brain to all parts of our body (see Figure 5). From the nervous system in our body spring voluntary and involuntary reactions to specific conditions.

A voluntary reaction is when we make a conscious decision to do something. Perhaps there is a pen lying on the table; our eyes pick up the light signals from it and the information is transmitted to the brain; the brain decides to pick up the pen and sends the message via specific nerves to the appropriate muscles of the arm and hand.

An involuntary reaction occurs, for example, if we touch a hot pan (see Figure 6). The heat sensors in the skin send an urgent warning message which, in this emergency situation, is dealt with by the spinal cord and a signal goes from here to the muscles of the arm to remove the hand from danger. At the same time a message goes up to the brain, which becomes aware of what is going on and prepares the body for further action. An involuntary reaction is also known as a reflex action.

There are other reflex actions which occur in the autonomic (involuntary or automatic) nervous system and, as the name suggests, these are carried out without our having any conscious knowledge about them, e.g., the heart continues beating without our telling it to all the time; similarly our digestive system keeps on working without direct orders continually from our conscious brain (which is very fortunate for

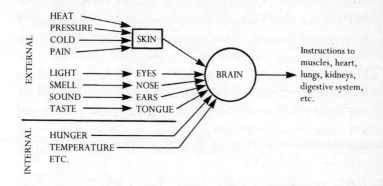

Figure 5. Transmitting information.

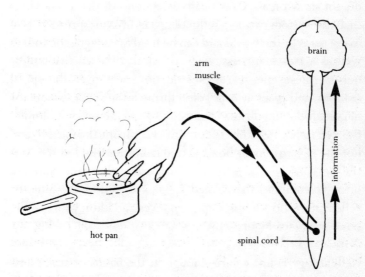

Figure 6. Involuntary reaction.

us!) All the reflexes mentioned above are well understood in Western society and can be found in medical textbooks.

The autonomic nervous system is characterized by a chain of little energy centres containing masses of nerve cells and there are several main groups of these in the body which are called plexuses. The coeliac (or solar) plexus is the largest and most 'responsive' plexus to consciousness, and it has a unique importance in that it is the centre of feelings and emotions. It is from here, under certain conditions, that quite pronounced and definite physical sensations of discomfort may be initiated.

### Reflexes in Reflexology – and How it Works

The reflexes which occur in reflexology are not the same as those within the nervous system. Not much is known scientifically about them – it is still very much an art and not a science – and as with the meridian lines in acupuncture they do not show on an X-ray or in dissection. All that is known is that the system works; reflexology is in widespread use in many parts of the world and can be used as a diagnostic tool as well as a treatment. Experience has also shown that unlike nerves, these energy reflexes do not cross over the spinal column, and react *without* going through the spinal connector nerves, following instead the body's zone lines. For example, the eye reflex in the left foot will react from the *left* eye and not the right as might be expected from the study of the central nervous system. Organs which are in the same zone are often related and the related reflex (as well as the affected reflex) may show a blockage, e.g., eyes and kidneys are in the same zone (see Figure 7).

Reflexology is not a cure, though in the hands of an experienced practitioner it can be very beneficial. Neither is it intended to provide a substitute for medical diagnoses or

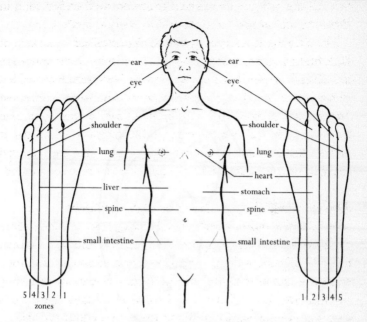

*Figure* 7. General relationship of body to foot area.

treatment. It is, however, extremely helpful and is without any of the side-effects which normally accompany conventional drugs and medicine. Success depends on the skill of the operator.

Reflex points are easiest to find in the feet, though they are to be found in other extremities of the body, i.e. hands, ears and tongue, as I said earlier. Each organ and muscle in the body is connected without crossing the spinal column by an energy pathway to a point in the foot (see Figure 7), hand, ear, etc. Pressure on these reflex points indicates the probable organs where there may be some disorder (not the *cause or nature* of the disorder – only that some disorder is there) and

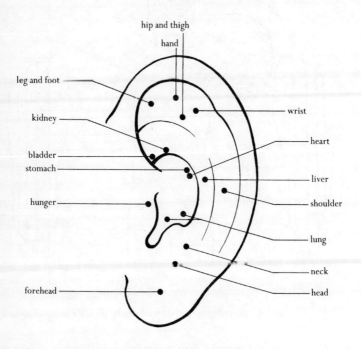

*Figure 8a*. Acupressure areas of the ear.

treatment then given brings about relaxation, as well as tend-
ing to normalize body conditions out of balance.

The most fascinating thing about these reflex points is that
they come to the surface in exactly the same relative position
as they are found in the body, and are most easily found on the
soles of the feet. If you imagine that with the feet close
together, looking at the soles, the big toes are the head, the
balls of the feet are the shoulders and down the centre is

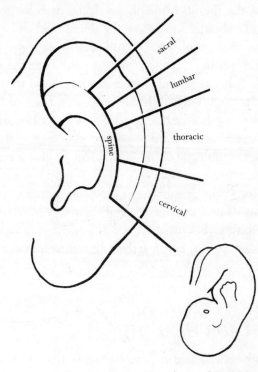

the ear reflects the shape
of the human embryo

*Figure 8b.* Acupressure points of the ear.

the spine – the curve of each foot here is even identical to the
side view of a person's back. The foot even narrows around
the waist area. Thus, all organs found above the waist in the
body are found above the waist of the foot, those positioned
below are found below. This shows that a basic knowledge of
anatomy is beneficial in reflexology and, indeed, the best
reflexologists could possibly be those with a medical or nurs-
ing background.

## *Thumb Technique*

The ball of the thumb is mainly used, the nails having been
filed down to about 2mm below the thumb pad and as pressure begins the thumb bends until almost at right angles,
relaxing and moving rather like a caterpillar over the area to
be treated. Other techniques are sometimes used to give the
best benefits, and if the reflex is not easily reached by one
method then another can be tried. Some practitioners use a
pencil for reaching awkward places, in order to give the pressure needed – too little being insufficient to give a reaction,
yet too much being painful.

Reflexology is not easily learnt by the lay person, so if you
want to carry out a treatment using the reflexes on the feet,
try Swiss Reflex Therapy (SRT); it is much easier to do and
its benefits are at least equal to those of reflexology (see chapter 5).

## *APPLIED KINESIOLOGY (TOUCH FOR HEALTH)*

Kinesiology is the scientific study of movement and posture.
Applied kinesiology (sometimes referred to as 'touch for
health') adapts the principles of kinesiology, combining them
in treatment with the meridian lines, to restore muscle balance, which is so important for good health and good posture.

As with reflexology, the treatment needs specialist study in
order to practise professionally; however, the diagnostic technique of touch for health is so simple – and so very interesting
– that I am including it in this chapter.

Like the diagnostic technique in reflexology, some aromatherapists use the diagnostic techniques of applied kinesiology before an aromatherapy treatment to find out as much
about their client's health as possible before selecting the

essential oils; the technique can also be used to discover if the essential oils selected are 'right' for the client.

One of the main ways it is used by complementary therapists of different disciplines is to discover if their client has an allergy to a particular food. It is an easy technique to learn and you can try it out on your partner or friend if you suspect they are eating or drinking something not good for their health; the system never lies!

I will start by telling you of my first experience with the technique. I was very sceptical when a friend of mine told me she could prove that white sugar was bad for the health. She asked me to hold out my arm, parallel to the floor, and asked me to push against her fingers when she put pressure on the back of my palm, to maintain the arm parallel to the floor. This was easy. She then told me that my muscles would not be able to hold my arm in this position if she asked me my name and I said 'Marjorie' instead of Shirley. She pressed very lightly and asked me my name. 'Marjorie' said I. She was pressing the back of my hand very lightly, but I could not maintain the parallel position – and though I resisted her pressure with all my might, my arm seemed to have no strength at all – and it fell to my side.

She repeated the exercise with me holding a small packet of white sugar in my hand and once more the arm fell to my side with her pressure. Holding an apple, however, I was able easily to resist her pressure, even when she increased it. I then tried it on my husband, with him holding the essential oils I had chosen for his asthma the previous year (I first tested him with a different name from his own). I asked if these essential oils were able to help his breathing – and he resisted easily, which meant that my oil choice had been a good one.

Treatment using applied kinesiology is not possible for the lay person; one has to attend a full course on the subject in order to put an ailing body back into balance. The diagnostic technique, however, is a great help to determine allergies, foods which may not be good for one or simply to verify the choice of essential oils before putting them in the bath!

## CONCLUSION

Aromatherapy is a treatment with essential oils; nothing more, nothing less. If you are interested in shiatsu, you can always learn more from a book on the subject; if you want to find out the state of health of your partner or friend, you can use the diagnostic technique adapted from reflexology on the reflexes of the feet; if you want to discover what should and should not be part of your daily food and drink intake (coffee is a good one to try!) or if you want to check your choice of essential oils to help your arthritis, kinesiology/touch for health is the thing to try.

And now – back to the subject of aromatherapy!

# chapter five

# SWISS REFLEX THERAPY (SRT)

Aromatherapists who want to practise reflexology as a treatment in its own right have to do further training. However, many practising aromatherapists use the reflex points (see Figures 9 and 10) for diagnostic purposes only; carried out before an aromatherapy treatment, together with a question and answer technique, this helps them select the right essential oils (it is not, however, intended to replace medical diagnosis or treatment). When the reflex points are used for this purpose, they are pressed only long enough to tell whether or not there is a disorder present – and all the bodily systems are covered in turn. As I have explained in the chapter on aromatherapy massage, many people have a natural talent for some practical subjects and although reflexology should only be done by trained therapists, it is possible to carry out Swiss Reflex Therapy (SRT for short) in the home.

SRT is a treatment technique I devised whilst in Switzerland in 1987 – hence the name! It is based on reflexology, though differing from it in several ways. I wanted to find a way of helping people to help themselves, using the reflexes every day, which would be easy for people to use on themselves (or each other) and which, if done conscientiously

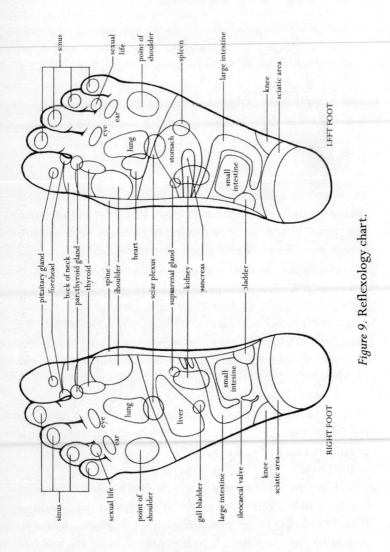

*Figure 9.* Reflexology chart.

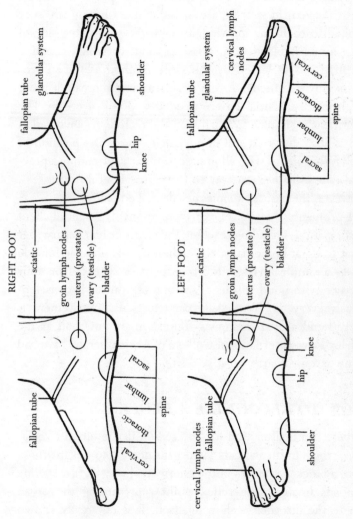

*Figure 10.* Reflex points on both sides of feet.

**every day**, would give faster results (and be less costly) than a weekly reflexology treatment.

With SRT, the reflexes explained in the previous chapter are massaged, in specific areas, rather than having pressure applied to each one individually with the ball or the side of the thumb. A bland cream base is used, to which is added essential oils (selected by the same method as for an aromatherapy treatment). A very small amount of cream is used, 30 drops of essential oil are needed in 30ml of cream. The treatment is simpler to learn than the techniques involved in reflexology, but it is still important to know the position of each reflex and as with all practical subjects, attending a practical course is the best way to learn (see Useful Addresses). However, the basic principles are described below.

A professional Swiss reflex treatment involves special client participation, including teaching the client or his/her partner what to do at home daily. Nevertheless, it is possible for you to do a simple Swiss reflex treatment on yourself or your partner with good results – so long as you do it conscientiously every day. With daily participation, improvement is fairly rapid – and therapists trained in this method at the Shirley Price International College of Aromatherapy have had some extraordinarily positive results.

## HOW TO RECOGNIZE A BLOCKAGE

If there is a malfunction for any reason in the blood circulation, which in turn affects the organs nearest to this malfunction, a blockage occurs in the energy pathway and crystalline deposits form at the reflex point representing the organ where the disorder is showing itself. It is not really known whether these deposits are in the blood circulation at the changeover from arteries to veins, or at the nerve endings.

But they can definitely be felt when they are present, and can certainly be broken down by correct pressure massage, bringing about relaxation plus a relief from the symptoms being suffered, by unblocking the energy flow.

The principle of good health is one of balance, when all bodily systems are behaving as nature intended, complementing one another to give the body this balance, or good health. The human body, apart from its more mysterious attributes, like the ability to think, is an intricate machine in which the blood acts like oil; therefore it is of prime importance to the working of that machine that the blood circulation flows unimpeded throughout the body. If there is congestion in the body the circulation is poor. If the circulation is upset by tension or stress then illness can occur, as the organs do not receive enough blood and nutrients (see Figure 11). Each cell is contracting and relaxing every moment, and when distress occurs this cannot be as regulated as it should be, and the healthy circulation is interfered with, resulting eventually in unhealthy organs. Every organ and every part of the body *needs* a correct flow of blood in order to be completely healthy.

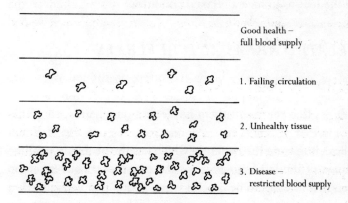

*Figure 11*. Circulation.

The blockage at a reflex point is always felt by someone when pressure is correctly applied. The feeling varies from a strange unpleasant feeling to a sharp knife-like pain or a gritty feeling, rather like bean bag filling (usually referred to as crystals) under the skin. This latter is the only reaction the operator can feel and for the other two he/she has to rely on feedback from questioning the person. Because of this, the operator's eyes should carefully watch the person's face, as well as their feet and a couple of minutes on each troubled reflex is usually enough at one treatment. Sometimes it is easier to detect the crystals when the thumb is made to glide over a small area with pressure. A good example of this is gliding from the reflex point of the bladder, up that of the ureter to the kidney reflex point, with pressure.

The first time a person experiences pressure on a reflex where there is a blockage the pain felt may be quite severe. This does not necessarily indicate a severe disorder and can sometimes be caused by tension in that person. It is a good idea, therefore, to commence all treatments, especially the first, with a series of preliminary general massage movements on the feet to induce a relaxed condition.

## RELATED AREAS AND REFLEXES

Just as organs in the body are often positioned over one another, or overlapping in some way, so therefore are the reflexes that represent them in the feet (and hands, etc.) This means that when there is a reaction, say, on the stomach reflex, it may be the pancreas which has the problem; similarly part of the left lung overlaps the heart, etc. Thus it can be seen that one has to be careful when asking people a question about a reaction, and even more careful when *replying* to the question, so as not to frighten them unnecessarily. Should the operator suspect there is something serious present, he should refer that person to his or her medical practitioner. Otherwise it is better to talk about general areas rather than specific points, and not to state exactly what one thinks may be the problem. The wonderful thing about SRT is that one can massage the whole tender area without risk of doing any harm and with beneficial results, even if one cannot pinpoint the exact organ requiring treatment.

Reflexes are related to one another and therefore if it is painful in the stomach area all the points in the digestive system should be treated; similarly if the kidney area shows a disorder, all organs connected with excretion should be treated.

## IMPORTANT POINTS TO REMEMBER

In Swiss Reflex Therapy the thumbs are the main 'tool' for carrying out the treatment, most movements being done with the side of the thumb in the form of a circle (it is absolutely essential that the thumb nails are very short, especially on the outer edge). Pressure applied is of the utmost importance, too little being insufficient to give a reaction on a tender reflex, yet too much being too painful on a tender one. The return half of the circle should always be light.

Always make certain that the person being treated is sitting comfortably or lying down as it is essential for him to be as relaxed as possible. The blood circulation is the key to all bodily functions and flows correctly only in a relaxed body. As I said before, when tension is present in an area that blood cannot flow through evenly; toxins are not removed fast enough and a disorder sets itself up.

Put both feet on a pillow on your knee and check that you, too, are in a comfortable position at a suitable height to reach the feet easily. You must also give complete concentration to what you are doing, with no other conscious thoughts; the diagnostic technique and the treatment following it must never be automatic but, as in all contact treatments, including aromatherapy, there must be total empathy between operator and recipient, and when this exists the healing energy flows from one to the other, making the benefits more satisfying and lasting.

The person being treated should be breathing in a slow, relaxed manner. Demonstrate to him/her how to take deep breaths, filling the lungs and slowly exhaling; breathe with your partner or friend until a comfortable rhythm is established. Then, with the person continuing with relaxed breathing, begin loosening up the muscles of the feet with a preliminary, relaxing foot massage, first wiping the feet with cotton wool and aromatherapy antiseptic toning lotion.

Please note that feet should always be held firmly, as it is both very irritating and contra to relaxation to have a light 'tickly' feeling on one's feet. This cannot be stressed enough, as a light touch can be very off-putting, however much one wants to try the treatment.

## Introductory Massage

1. Holding foot firmly, rotate ankle clockwise then anti-clockwise slowly twice each way.
2. Rotate big toe twice each way.
3. With thumbs overlapped, zig-zag down sole of foot from toes to heel, then press firmly all the way up, keeping thumbs sideways.
4. With thumbs on sole of foot, and fingers on top, gently twist foot to the left, then to the right to spread the toes.
5. Using whole hand, massage round ankle bone.
6. Using palm of hand, stroke firmly down inner side of sole.

7. Wrap the foot in a towel to keep warm.
8. Repeat 1–7 on the other foot.

You are now ready to start the diagnostic procedure (this part is not a treatment!) – and remember that as you are looking at the soles of the feet in front of you, the right foot is on your LEFT and the left foot is on your RIGHT (see Figure 9 on page 54).

## CLIENT PARTICIPATION – QUESTIONS!

Participation by the person being treated is an integral and essential part of both the assessment and the treatment.

### Assessment questions:

As you locate and gently press a reflex, watch the person's face carefully for a reaction. If there is not one, you should ask a negative question:

'So you don't have any respiratory difficulties?' (when pressing the lung reflex)

'So you don't have backache very often?' (when pressing the spinal reflexes)

'So you don't suffer from stress?' (when pressing the solar plexus reflex)

The answer will probably be 'No'. However, some people have a stronger pain threshold than others (or you may not have been quite in the right place), so they may say 'Actually, I do!' This kind of negatively phrased question is less worrying than asking all the time 'Do you have a problem with …?' followed by the representative reflex being pressed. If, however, you can feel grittiness or the person's face screws up, the question should be positive:

'Ah! So you suffer with backache' or

'H'mm! Your reaction suggests (or my fingers can feel) that you may have problem connected with your lungs'

The person can usually tell you what the problem is; however, if they are not aware of one, tell them that they probably have just an imbalance in that area – which is precisely what it is.

### Treatment questions:

During the assessment, using the reflexes as a diagnostic tool, you should have discovered the person's pain threshold, so adjust your pressure accordingly. Having found the pain threshold, maintain the same pressure throughout the treatment of that reflex area. Every now and again you ask:

'Has the pain reduced at all yet?'

After about half a minute of massage, the person will say incredulously, 'Yes, it's not as painful – are you pressing as hard as you were before?' Having assured them you are you now say:

'I want you to tell me when the pain has gone.' Then –

'Has it gone yet?'

When the pain has gone, treatment on that reflex is finished for that day and you move on to the next one.

When people are stressed, be aware that all points may be very sensitive, so be gentle at first, until you assess their pain threshold. Even if they have told you their particular problem (or problems), still carry out a full analysis to check related organs. It is best to work through each system of the body, completing wherever possible one system on both feet before beginning on the next. This not only keeps up the continuity of related reflexes but also is better than breaking off in the middle of the digestive system, say at the stomach, and starting again a few minutes after treating another reflex, e.g. kidney, on the way down the foot; it also helps maintain equilibrium and relaxation induced in the body. (There are, of course, exceptions to every rule, and, as an example, it is easier to find the adrenal gland reflex when one has found the kidney reflex while doing the excretory system.)

For the diagnostic technique, the reflex points of each system should be found on *both* feet before going on to the next one (the digestive system is more complicated and full instructions are given in the order of work). Don't forget to note which reflexes have an uncomfortable reaction and therefore which systems of the body need a treatment.

The following text goes through the order of work for the diagnostic technique, showing how to hold the foot when locating some of the points. Use it together with the questioning technique describe above.

The following text goes through the order of work for the diagnostic technique, showing how to hold foot when locating some of the points. Use it together with the assessment questions described above.

## *DER OF WORK*

1. **Nervous system:**

   Solar plexus     — just under ball of foot, in centre (see Figure 12).

   Sciatic nerve     — (See Figure 10.)

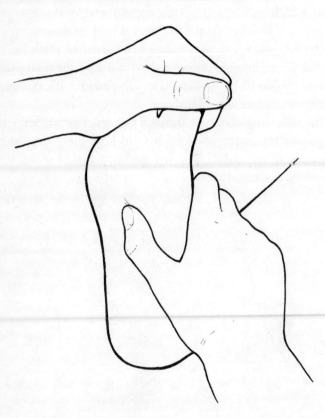

*Figure 12.* Solar plexus reflex.

2. **Glandular system:**

Pituitary gland     — lower part of big toe cushion, in centre

Parathyroid       ⎫    — these two are very close to one
                     ⎬      another;

Thyroid           ⎭      thyroid usually treated as an area

Sex gland           — just under cushion of fourth toe

Adrenal gland     — top inside edge of kidney — best to
                              do this reflex when doing kidney
                              (see Figure 16).

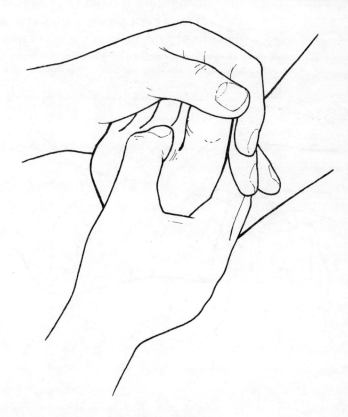

*Figure 13.* Eye Reflex.

3. **Sinuses, Eye and Ear:**

Sinuses                    — centre of cushion in four small toes.

Eye                        — between second and third toe *above* ball of foot, just *below* neck of toe (see Figure 13).

Ear                        — same as above, but between fourth and fifth toes.

4. **Bone and muscular system:**

Spine                      — from big toe (cervical) to heel (coccyx) on inner edge of foot. Curve of foot relates to curve regions of spine (See Figure 14).

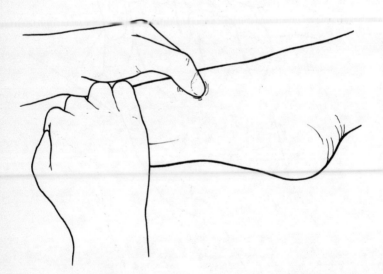

*Figure 14.* Part of the spine reflex.

Neck   — all round big toe neck (see Figure 15).

Shoulder   — main shoulder blade area found in fleshy part under big toe. Extremity of shoulder found just below neck of little toe.

Hip and knee   — follow diagram on page 54 (approximately on same level as bladder reflex but on little toe side of foot).

## 5. **Respiratory system:**

Lungs   — large area on centre of ball of foot (see diagram page 54).

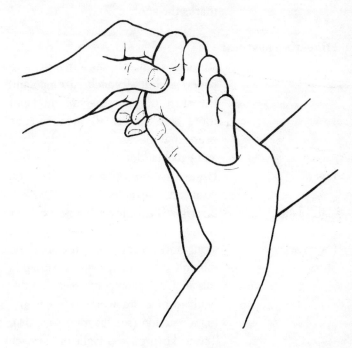

*Figure 15*. Neck reflex.

6. **Excretory system:**

Kidney — below solar plexus and slightly toward inside of foot. Kidney is easier to find if bladder is found first, then slide thumb up and slightly inwards on ureter tube until kidney reflex is felt. (see Figure 16).

(Adrenal gland is on top inside edge of kidney).

Ureter — narrow area between kidney and bladder.

Bladder — located on inside of foot near heel. Very often a little raised area on foot marks the spot.

7. **Digestive system:**

— stomach is mostly on left foot, also pancreas, but stomach entrance and the start of pancreas are on right foot, and this small area can be pressed if necessary after the liver and gall-bladder.

Liver — large area on outside of foot, on your left hand side.

Gall-bladder — on right hand lower edge of liver then move to foot on right hand side.

Pancreas — along bottom edge of stomach reflex.

Stomach — difficult, as so many organs overlap in this area. No problem to *treat*, but difficult to pinpoint which reflex is giving a reaction (see diagram page 54). Try to keep on top right of stomach reflex.

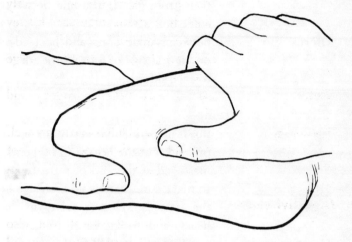

*Figure 16*. Kidney reflex.

Small intestine    – below waist of foot – middle to inside edge; foot on your right first, then move to foot on your left.

Ileocaecal valve    – still on your left, move towards large intestine.

Large intestine    – carefully work upwards and along to waist of foot. Remember that as you pass kidney a reaction from *that* reflex may be felt. Continue across on to other foot, and complete.

8. **Reproductive system:**

Ovaries                    — between ankle bone and heel edge
                             on little toe side of foot.
Fallopian Tube             — approximately 1cm further up foot
                             than groin gland, in a line between
                             ankle bones.
Uterus                     — between ankle bone and heel edge
                             on big toe side of foot. Work a little
                             to each side also.

9. **Circulatory system:**

                           — this is helped with every reflex point
                             pressed, but the heart can be gently
                             massaged at the end of a treatment
                             to make sure there is no blockage in
                             the arteries, veins or valves in the
                             heart, and to increase circulation.
Heart                      — usually found on left foot (right fac-
                             ing you) above and slightly to the left
                             of the solar plexus.
Spleen                     — top right hand edge of stomach reflex.
Lymphatic system           — follow diagram (page 54) and cover
                             all lymphatic points on each foot.
                             *Note:* The spleen and lymphatic sys-
                             tem are included here because of
                             their close relationship to the blood.

By the time you are finished the client assessment the person
should be well relaxed and ready to receive Swiss Reflex
Therapy on the problem areas.

## *TREATMENT OF TROUBLED REFLEXES*

It is best now to work through each system of the body, rather than one foot at a time (as in the diagnostic technique on page 61), completing wherever possible one system on both feet before beginning on the next. This not only keeps up the continuity of related reflexes but also is better than breaking off in the middle of the digestive system and completing it a few minutes later after finishing that foot; it also helps maintain equilibrium and relaxation induced in the body.

1. Starting on the left foot, apply a very small amount of cream over the whole of the foot.
2. With the hands facing opposite ways but close together (see Figure 30 on page 99) place them so that the palms are on the top of the foot. Massage up to the ankle only, returning as in Figure 31 on page 99, sandwiching the foot firmly.
3. Repeat several times, then wrap in a towel.
4. Repeat numbers 1 and 2 on the right foot and begin the treatment on this foot.

    N.B. A treatment always begins with the solar plexus reflex area and finishes on the kidney/bladder area.
5. Hold the right foot with your left hand and begin by massaging the whole of the solar plexus reflex area with the whole of the length of your right thumb. Do this in a circular motion as firmly as the tolerance of the individual person will allow (if he or she is highly stressed even a gentle stroking will seem painful). Keep circling at the tolerance level, maintaining the same pressure (to give *slight* discomfort) while asking the person to tell you if he or she feels it is easing. Keep circling until the person is able to tell you that the discomfort has completely

gone. If it is still painful after one minute, the original pressure was obviously too strong and the movement should be repeated with just enough pressure to take the person to his or her lowest pain threshold.

6. Massage (in circular movements as described above) any reflex areas which presented a problem during the diagnostic technique e.g. the lung area for bronchial problems, digestive system area for constipation (concentrating on the large intestine reflex area, in a clockwise direction) and spinal areas for backache, muscular aches and pains, rheumatism or arthritis. Change your hand positions when necessary. For a long area like the spine, do a small circle at a time, moving down a little and repeating until the whole length of the spine has been covered.

7. When all troubled bodily systems have been covered, place your right hand across your body and placing it over the person's toes, massage in a firm elongated circle, following the kidney-ureter-bladder; massage with pressure from kidney to bladder, relaxing the pressure on the return half of the circle.

8. Repeat numbers 1 and 2 and re-wrap in the towel.

9. Repeat movements 4–7 on the left foot, reversing 'right' and 'left' in the text. In a professional treatment the therapist would then ask the client or carer to carry out the same treatment (without the diagnostic technique) with the therapist's help, to be sure that the treatment would be done on the correct areas and with the correct pressure. It would then be emphasised that the treatment had to be done every day for the best results.

# chapter six

# SIMPLE AROMATHERAPY TREATMENT TECHNIQUES

Before I explain the various treatment techniques possible with aromatherapy, I should like to point out a very important fact. We are all aware that any *one* form of treatment is not always totally effective on any one person, for any one particular problem, when used completely on its own.

For *some* people in certain circumstances and for *some* problems – yes – one form of treatment can succeed. But we must remember that it is not always as straightforward as that. Some people respond better to aromatherapy when combined with Swiss Reflex Therapy (see page 53); others when they complement the massage treatment with home use of the essential oils in the bath. Some will benefit completely using only oils in the bath – others will not.

So we must have a sensible approach to the use of this important and interesting therapy and combine it with other therapies as and where necessary.

The easiest ways of using essential oils to help any disorder are:

- inhaling them.
- putting them in the bath.
- using them in a compress.

- applying them to the body, or part of the body, in a carrier oil or lotion (for massage).
- taking them internally (see Author's Note on page vii).

### *Internally:*

Daily ingestion of true essential oil guarantees proper balance and functioning of intestines, and fights internal infections. It must be emphasized that poor quality or perfume quality essential oils should never be taken internally. Genuine essential oils can play a major role in the prevention of many diseases, including cancer. Aromatologists and some French doctors prescribe essential oils to be taken internally, either in a special dispersant or to be taken with honey and water. My friend's mother, who lives in Aix-en-Provence in France, is treated *only* by an aromatherapy doctor and wouldn't go back to drugs and tablets. The only thing is, she says, it tastes like medicine, because essential oils are so concentrated!

It is exceptionally important, however, not only to know which essential oils can be taken internally, but also to be sure that they are purchased from a reliable source. Unfortunately as aromatherapy becomes more well known, many more people are selling 'aromatherapy' oils, but ONLY true, genuine distilled or expressed essential oil is suitable for internal use.

The following oils should not be taken internally at all:

- absolutes, such as jasmine or rose
- resins, such as benzoin

Appropriate genuine essential oils, obtained by distillation and procured from a reliable source, can be taken as medicine, provided the correct dose is given. Never exceed 2 or 3 drops (suitably diluted) 3 times a day and take them only on five days out of seven – Saturdays and Sundays are the easiest ones to miss out! These two days without oils gives your system a short rest period each week before recommencing treatment, if it is necessary to do so. However, teas made with essential oils can be drunk daily, as the quantity of essential oil actually consumed in these is so small.

If you decide to ingest oils, then the honey and water method is probably the easiest. For this, take one teaspoonful of runny honey and add 1-3 drops (in total) of the chosen essential oil or oils. Stir well to dissolve the oils, then add 1-2 teaspoons of boiling water. Stir again and swallow. If you are very brave, just drop the essential oil on to a sugar lump and eat it! You should have 2 to 3 doses per day, depending on your problem.

Another way of taking oils internally is by making a 'tea', using tea bags and essential oil. This too, can be taken 2 to 3 times per day. Experiment with different 'flavours', choosing carefully from the oils you need.

Make a pot of tea using one tea bag only, and add 2 drops of essential oil. After 2 minutes, stir, remove tea bag and pour a cupful. I prefer these teas without milk or sugar, but sugar can be added if preferred. If milk *has* to be used, the tea must be made with 2 tea bags and then follow the instructions as for one bag.

Almost any essential oil can be used. Follow the therapeutic index on page 182, mixing two or three essential oils together in a small dropper bottle to be used as required, when you find a mixture you like.

By the way, Earl Grey tea is just ordinary tea with essential oil of bergamot in it, and I often put 2 drops of bergamot into my teapot if I have no Earl Grey tea!

The following is only a selection of the ailments which can be treated internally:

| coughs and colds | headaches and painful periods |
| flatulence | cystisis |
| indigestion | depression |
| constipation | stones in the kidney or |
| diarrhoea | urinary tract. |

## *Inhalations:*

This is one of the best ways of using essential oils therapeutically.

One of the easiest ways to inhale essential oils is simply to put about 4-8 drops on a paper towel or handkerchief and breathe in very deeply (through the nose if possible) two or three times. Put one on your pillow, beside your nose, at nights – with nasal congestion or asthma it is an ideal way to ensure a free breathing passage during the night.

Another way of inhaling is to put essential oils into hot water and breathe the vapour which comes from it. This time only 2-4 drops of essential oil should be put in 100ml of hot water. It is best to put a towel over your head and the basin, to keep the vapour in a small area. Breathe in (preferably through the nose) until the aroma has almost disappeared. This treatment should be repeated 3 times a day. (Not suitable for asthmatics, who should use the dry inhalation method above.)

Madame Maury used inhalations for her clients between aromatherapy massage treatments and found it successful for many of the complaints brought to her salon.

Inhalations are mainly used for:

| tension | headaches |
| disorder relating to the respiratory tract, e.g., | |
| colds | sore throat |
| blocked sinuses | cough, etc. |
| asthma (without steam) | |

### Foot and Hand Baths:

This treatment is a nice easy one to do while sitting down at night. All that is needed is a bowl of hand-hot water with 6 to 8 drops of essential oil. Keep a kettle of just-boiled water beside the bowl to add to the water if it goes too cool. Steep hands or feet for 10 to 15 minutes, moving them around every now and again. Wrap in a dry towel after soaking, and leave for another 15 minutes. Finish the treatments by massaging into your feet and lower legs a little massage oil containing some essential oils. (See pages 114–119.)

Troubles which benefit best with a bath treatment are:

| | |
|---|---|
| rheumatism | dermatitis |
| arthritis | dry skin, etc. |

### Baths:

The bath should be hand-hot before adding the essential oils and 4 drops in ½ bath of water, 8 in ¾ bath of water, are all that are needed. One should stay in the bath for at least 10 minutes, turning over if possible half way through. (Not necessary when water completely covers body.) Essential oil baths are very pleasant to have, and most beneficial. N.B. Swish water well to disperse oil.

I always add my essential oil undiluted, as described above, but some people like to mix them into something to help disperse the oils more easily. An often recommended method is to add them to a vegetable carrier oil, but when I tried it, I found that after a while, the plug chain became discoloured and in any case, the bath was much more difficult to clean, as it gets an oily mark all round it. One of the best mediums to use is a teaspoon of dried milk; add your essential oils to it and then make it into a thin paste with water, just as you would with custard. You can also mix your choice of oils with a couple of teaspoons of yoghurt or pouring cream. Whichever medium you use, after adding to the bath swish well, to disperse mixture fully.

By the way, do not use resins or absolutes in a plastic bath unless you dilute them as above; because they are denser than essential oils, they sink to the bottom and if not thoroughly dispersed, the residual solvent will make a permanent mark on your bath.

Conditions benefiting from baths:

| | |
|---|---|
| insomnia | menstruation problems |
| nervous tension | coughs and colds |
| muscular disorders | headaches |
| circulation problems | fluid retention, etc. |

## *Compresses:*
Very useful as a treatment for skin problems, bruises, muscular and chest pains, and indeed can be used over a problem area for disorders such as painful periods.

The normal strength for a compress to cover an area of about 6" square is about 5 or 6 drops in 100ml water as for inhalations, but I have used 2 or 3 drops neat on a piece of damp gauze for a bad bruise with excellent results.

Old sheeting in four thickness (or an old handkerchief) is ideal for a compress, cut large enough to cover the area being treated. Do not use *medicated* lint of gauze, but untreated cotton wool in the roll can be used for small areas. However, remember that cotton wool is more absorbent than sheeting and will probably soak up more liquid, so do bear this, and the size of the compress, in mind when mixing essential oils. For example 200ml with 8 drops may be needed for a large area, but a small area may only take 50ml of water, and 3 or 4 drops of essential oil. The concentration of oil onto or into the body is what counts therapeutically, as will be seen later when oils are mixed for massage.

Pour enough measured hot water into a bowl to be soaked up in the size of compress chosen for the treatment (experiment and practice will soon make it easy to determine the quantity necessary) and add essential oils chosen from the Therapeutic Index on page 182.

Put the compress into the water and essential oils, and squeeze out so that it will not drip, but not enough to make it nearly dry.

Place a compress over the area being treated, and wrap a sheet of clingflim around it. To help the compress to work more efficiently put a pre-warmed towel and blanket over the top to keep the compress warm. Ideally, leave on for two hours (at least). For the back, apply a compress in reverse order; warm towel on bed, then plastic sheet, then compress; and then lie on it and cover the top of the body with a warm blanket.

Occasionally, and for a tiny area, a compress using neat essential oils is very beneficial, for example, sprains, bruises, wounds, neuralgia, abscesses, etc. Here, the neat oil is put onto the area and can be covered with a damp gauze or cotton wool, which can then be kept on the skin by the use of micropore surgical tape or clingfilm.

Conditions benefiting best from compresses are:

| | |
|---|---|
| skin problems | painful periods |
| neuralgia | sprains |
| bruises | muscular aches and pains |
| open wounds | |

Neat essential oils are also very beneficial in an emergency such as a burn, nettle rash, scald or insect bite to ease the initial discomfort and act as an antiseptic. In these cases they do not need to be covered; just apply neat essential oil at regular intervals and leave. *Herpes simplex* (i.e. cold sores), though not an emergency, responds wonderfully to neat application of essential oil. N.B. Do not go into the sun or use a sunbed immediately afterwards if citrus oils are used, especially berg-amot.

## Gargling:

To help a sore throat or prevent a cold from going onto the chest, gargling is an excellent method of using essential oils. Add three drops of essential oil to 1 tsp. of alcohol (eg vodka) and make up to ½ cup with water. Stir before each mouthful.

Conditions benefiting from gargling:

sore throat                              virus infections
coughs

## Self-application (embrocation):

This simply means the putting on of essential oils by yourself – or by a third party (i.e. a carer) without involving massage or an aromatherapist. It is a very successful, inexpensive and easy way of helping (daily, if necessary) localized complaints like arthritis, rheumatism, chest disorders, digestive and menstrual pain and many other problems.

The proportions of essential oil to be diluted in the carrier are the same as for massage – 15-30 drops in 50ml of veg-etable carrier or a non-greasy base lotion, made by emulsify-ing oil and water together. The latter method is much more suitable for self-application, as it does not stain any clothing put on straight afterwards and leaves the skin with a silky, but non-slip, feel to it.

## Massage:

This is the most useful form of aromatherapy and gives great benefit to almost any condition. Being so important, the next two chapters are devoted to this subject.

# chapter seven

# AN EXPLANATION
# OF MASSAGE

The field of massage has widened considerably over the last 10·
to 20 years, incorporating new types of massage such as shiatsu and reflexology, although these last two are mainly con-
cerned with *pressure* rather than *massage* as we understand it.

In body massage pressure is, of course, used, but in many
different ways. The nearest movement in a Western massage
to shiatsu and reflexology pressure is the first part only of
what we call thumb frictions, where pressure is put on certain
parts of the body, with the thumbs, before making small circles over that area.

The word 'massage' comes from the Greek word meaning
*to knead*, and it is one of the oldest forms of treatment for
human ailments. Hippocrates (460–380 BC) said about a dis-
located shoulder, '... it is necessary to rub the shoulder gently
and smoothly with soft hands. The physician must be experienced in many things, but assuredly also in rubbing.' Various
systems and techniques have been developed over the years
and people with many and varied qualifications have prescribed and performed massage.

The effects of massage treatment naturally depend greatly
upon the technical skill and knowledge of the masseur or
masseuse. Through proper and skilful massage all the functions

of the organs of the body – skin, muscles, nerves, glands, etc. – are stimulated, and by the increased circulation of the blood and lymph, the clearing away of body waste is assisted.

Body massage movements can vary from soft, light, rhythmical stroking movements designed to relax the muscles and nerves, to heavy pounding and kneading designed to break up fatty areas.

In aromatherapy we use mostly stroking movements, or effleurage as it is called, a little kneading and some frictions (called compression), and it is well to understand these before trying to help anyone.

## EFFLEURAGE

(a) Superficial stroking: used always in the return direction from deep stroking, but can be used on its own. Over large areas the palms (and fingers) of the hand are used and they should relax to the shape of the body underneath them, in other words, mould themselves to the part of the body being massaged.

(b) Deep stroking: this is done with the whole hand as in superficial stroking, but it is done with pressure and always in the direction of the heart. (This helps the venous flow.) It is only done in that direction, the return journey always being a light, superficial stroke.

When doing effleurage, the hands should keep in contact with the body all the time, and the rhythm of the strokes should be slow and even.

Effleurage improves the venous flow, i.e., helps to remove congestion in the veins. Because of this fresh blood can circulate more freely, taking nutrients to all organs through which it passes. The absorption of waste products is hastened and the lymphatic circulation improved. As an added bonus, it is extremely soothing and relaxing, particularly for nervous, irritated or over-tired people.

## COMPRESSION

(a) Petrissage (or kneading). This is when a muscle, part of a muscle group is picked up and squeezed or rolled, then released while the other hand moves to the adjacent area to repeat the process. This movement is usually done with both hands, using the palm and the whole length of the fingers, or the thumb and fingers, depending on the size of the muscle area being massaged. It is essential that this movement is carried out only after the area has been previously relaxed by effleurage, and it should be slow, gentle and rhythmical, always returning to starting point without a break in contact or with a superficial stroke.

Petrissage increases the circulation and the removal of waste products, thus helping fatigue. The skin, deep and superficial or 'surface' tissues are all stimulated into further activity. The sudden releasing of the stretched muscle fibres causes them to contract momentarily, thus strengthening them, and finally, fat and fibrous tissues can sometimes be broken down.

(b) Frictions (or deep rubbing in circles). These movements can be carried out with the palm of the hand, the cushions of the thumbs or one or more fingers. With frictions, it is as though the part of the hand being used is 'stuck' to the skin on the body being massaged: the skin must move, *with* the part of the hand being used, *over* the tissues beneath, with pressure. After several circles over one area have been completed, the pressure is released so that the hand (*without losing contact*) can glide to the next area and the movement be repeated. Pressure must be firm but not cause injury to the underlying tissues.

Frictions aid the removal of excess fluid in the body and stimulate the circulation. Most importantly, they can sometimes break down fat, fibrous thickening and tension nodules in the part being treated.

There is another form of body massage used called **percussion** which, as the name suggests, is made up of short, sharp movements. There are many types of percussion (with names like pounding, hacking, cupping, etc!) but none of them are used in aromatherapy, as none are relaxing.

You can see how important it is for massage movements to be done correctly, and how the best results are obviously obtained by visiting a qualified masseur. However, as in all arts, such as cooking, painting, pottery, etc., certain people without professional training possess a natural ability to carry out these arts, and with just a little help, to make sure the technique is correct, these people can attain quite a good standard. It is for *this type of person* that I have given such a detailed description of the massage movements. They will, with the assistance of essential oils, be able to help their relatives and friends in a completely natural and harmless way, with no risk of side effects.

## REMINDERS

Massage stimulates the blood circulation and all the systems in the body, so do not treat anyone who:

- has just finished a meal or is needing food!
- is at the beginning of a heavy period
- is under heavy sedation or on a lot of tablets (except gently here, as usually this type of person will benefit from treatment)

- has an infection of any sort, or if there is a fracture in the
  area

Massage *gently* and carefully over recent scar tissue and varicose veins, both of which can be helped by choosing the right
essential oils and using only effleurage, to aid the penetration
of the oils. (Both conditions can be harmed by heavy and
incorrect massage techniques.)

During pregnancy massage is recommended on any part of
the body up to the fourth or fifth month. After this time it
would not be comfortable to lie face downwards, so only
massage areas which do not involve this position.

Do not massage heavily over bruised or broken skin, but do
treat these with essential oils either by a compress or very
lightly applying neat oils into the affected area.

# chapter eight

# AROMATHERAPY MASSAGE TECHNIQUES

Always make sure that the room you are working in is warm, and that your nails are short. Many small area massage treatments, like shoulders, can be done in the living room, but if you are wanting to cover the whole back, or legs, then a firm bed in a warm bedroom is essential. Better still, use a table with blankets or a strip of foam for comfort.

I will start with back massage; it is the longest and most complicated, but it is the easiest to practise the movements on a larger area, and having become familiar with the basic movements, you will find it easier to adapt for special smaller tension areas. Miss out all the numbers with * beside them to start with, and add these as you become more proficient and confident.

It is important that the person being massaged is breathing out whenever spinal pressures are being done (see figure 20), also for massage on the abdomen, which also involves pressure. The breathing should only be adjusted, and be quite normal, not exaggerated.

Choose the essential oils needed and mix them in a 50ml bottle of blended carrier oils (grapeseed or almond, with calendula, wheatgerm or avocado if needed), as explained in Chapter 9.

## BACK MASSAGE

1.  Put about a teaspoon of massage oil in the palm of one hand. Rub both hands together lightly, then spread the oil over the whole back with wide sweeping effleurage movements.

2.  Put hands at the base of the spine, fingers facing the opposite shoulder all the time; and stroke firmly up each side of the spine, using the whole hand, round the shoulder blade, then very lightly down the sides of the back to the base of the spine. Repeat 4 or 5 times. (See Figure 17.)

3.  Put one hand over the other (reinforced hand) to give strength to the next movement – still at the base of the

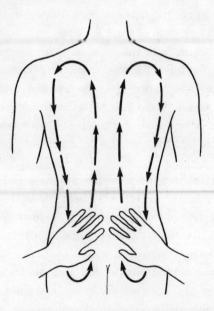

*Figure 17.* Movement 2 (back).

spine. Push firmly up one side of the back to the shoulder area, where the hands cross the spine upwards between the shoulder blades, go right round the shoulder, cross the spine upwards and go right round the other shoulder, making a figure eight 4 or 5 times, bringing the hands back to the base of the spine on the last repeat. During this movement keep the *whole* of the reinforced hand on the body. (See Figures 18 and 19.)

4.* Pressures down spinal channels (with rhythmic breathing). As you cross the spine for the last time in No. 3 (going away from you) turn your hands and place both thumbs together and facing one another in the spinal channel at the left side of the spine (about 1 or 2cm from the spine itself). Press firmly down with thumbs

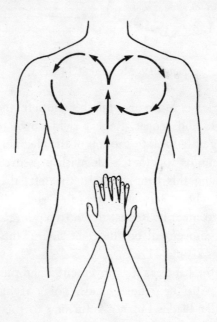

*Figure 18.* Movement 3 (back).

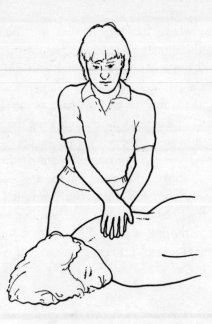

*Figure 19.* Movement 3 (back).

and release. Move one thumb's width further down the channel and repeat. Repeat right down to hip level. Slide gently back to the top of the channel, and, keeping thumbs together, slide with pressure (no special breathing this time) first to the left, then the right thumb about 2cm at a time, i.e., slide left and bring right to meet it. Repeat down to hip level. Repeat the whole movement on the right side of the spine. (See Figures 20 and 21.)

5.  Place the hands as for movement 2 and push firmly up back with the whole hands, going right round the shoulder blades but not returning to the base of the spine. Go round the shoulder blades again, this time

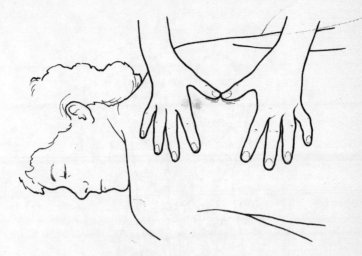

*Figure 20*. Movement 4 (back) showing position of thumbs
in one spinal channel (one thumb facing head, one thumb
facing feet)

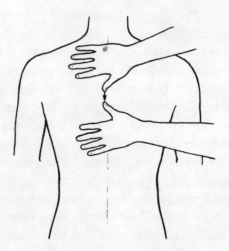

*Figure 21*. Movement 4 (back).

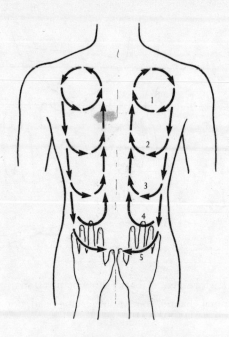

*Figure 22.* Movement 5 (back).

finishing the circle a little lower down the back. Repeat the shoulder blade circle, finishing even lower this time. just above waist level. Repeat, finishing a little lower down each time until the last circle finishes at the base of the spine, having covered the whole of the back in one circle. (See Figure 22.)

6. Place the hands as for movement 2 and push straight up the back over the tops of shoulders with pressure, returning very lightly and without pressure. Repeat twice.

7. Push up the back and out towards the armpits with pressure, returning by the same path but without pressure. Repeat twice.

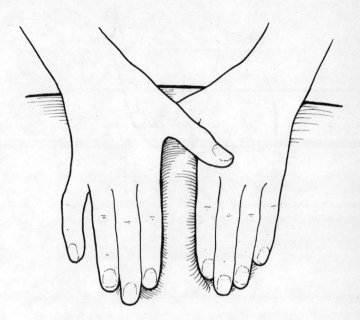

*Figure 23.* Movement 9 (back).

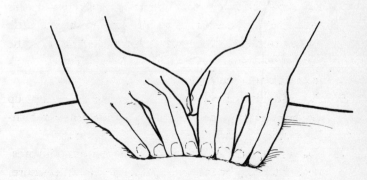

*Figure 24.* Movement 10 (back).

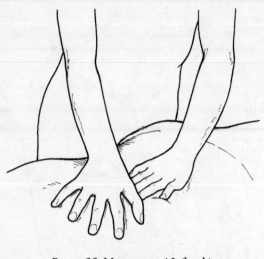

*Figure 25*. Movement 12 (back).

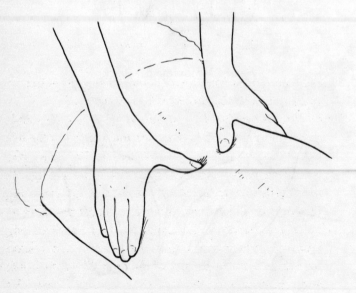

*Figure 26*. Movement 13 (back).

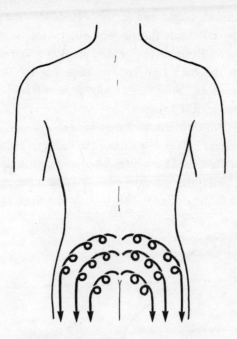

*Figure 27.* Movement 13 (back).

8. Push up the back and out to the chest with pressure, returning lightly as before. Repeat twice.

9.* Do the first half of the movement no. 2 up the shoulders and turn the fingers to face the armpit on the left side. Let the thumbs overlap as the finger lengths squeeze together and release once, quickly and lightly, moving their length towards the armpit and repeating the squeeze and release. Move and repeat twice. Now move one hand's width down the back, and starting again near the spine, repeat the squeeze and release four times towards the side of the body. Move the hands and repeat once more at waist level. (See Figure 23.)

10. Slide back to the top of the spine and place the finger

pads in a *straight* line in the left spinal channel. Press firmly and push the fingers out to the armpits with pressure. Return very gently, moving one hand's width down the back and repeat. (See Figure 24.) Repeat twice more. Now repeat movements 9 and 10 on the right side of the back.

11. Repeat movement no. 2 four times.
12.*Effleurage up the left side of the back, from hip level to the shoulders. Using alternate hands, push up with fingers facing the shoulders at the spine side, moving out towards the side of the body (opening the fingers as you

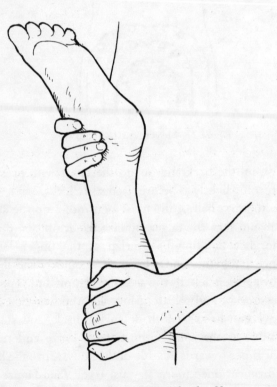

*Figure 28.* Movement 3 (back of leg).

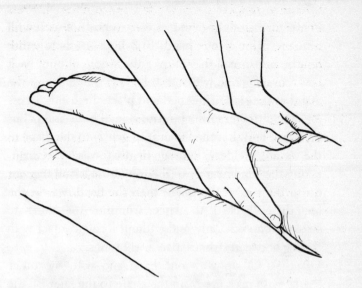

*Figure 29.* Movement 4 (back of leg).

do so). The next hand comes underneath the first one and repeats the movement; each hand moves up the body a little as well as going sideways like a fan. Finish at the shoulder with the hand nearest the head while the other comes in again at hip level to start again. Repeat three times. Repeat the whole movement on the right side. (See Figure 25.)

13. Using the thumbs, do friction circles from the waist on either side of the spine, out and round the hip bone. Repeat three times, each time doing a smaller curve. (See Figures 26 and 27.)

14. Repeat movement no. 2 four or five times.

## THE BACK OF THE LEGS

1.  Put a small amount (about ½ teaspoonful) of mixed oil into the palm of one hand. Rub both hands together lightly, and spread the oil over the whole of both back legs (covering one with a towel).

2.  Stand at the side of the bed and place the hands across one ankle (fingers facing out to side of body and palms on top of leg). Let the fingers fall gently to the shape of the leg at the side. Effleurage firmly towards the thigh, taking the hand nearest to the top of the leg all the way up to the top of the thigh; then the hand nearest the feet to the back of the knee. Continue this alternate stroking one way only, and without losing contact with the leg between strokes, five or six times.

3.  Lift the foot up with one hand and with the other stroke with pressure from the ankle to the knee on the back of the leg, keeping the palm in the centre and the fingers relaxed round the leg. Repeat four or five times. (See Figure 28.)

4.  Stand at the bottom of the bed and slide the thumbs up the leg from the ankle to the knee firmly, with pressure, and return with light effleurage down the sides of the leg. (See Figure 29.)

5.  Repeat movement 2 five or six times.

6.  Repeat all the movements on the other leg.

## FRONT OF THE LEGS

1.  Put oil on as before.

2.  With the hands facing opposite ways but close together, effleurage firmly up the whole of the leg and lightly return down the sides, sandwiching the foot as shown. Repeat three or four times, finishing with an extra half

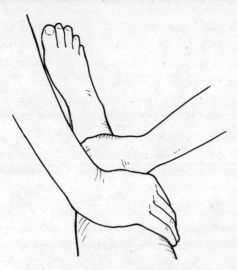

*Figure 30*. Movement 2a (front of leg).

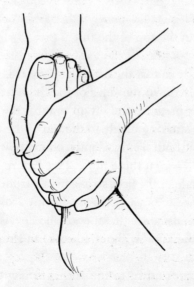

*Figure 31*. Movement 2b (front of leg).

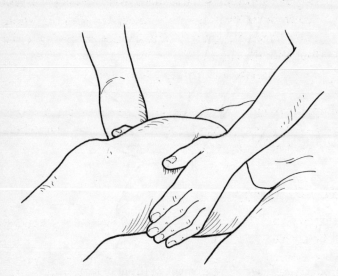

*Figure 32*. Movement 3 (front of leg).

movement to the top of the thigh. (See Figures 30 and 32.)

3.  Turn the body so that the hands face towards the ankle, stroke lightly down the sides of the thigh to the knee. There, apply pressure and lift up towards the middle of the top leg, stroking firmly to the top of the thigh with the whole of both hands. Gently return down sides of the thigh and repeat three times. (See Figure 32.)

4.  Facing the side of the bed, stroke firmly from inside the leg at the knee to outside, diagonally upwards and using alternate hands until the top of the leg is reached. Return to the knee without a break, and repeat three or four times.

5.  Bring the hands down to the knee, turning them (and you) to face upwards, and make a bridge of your first

fingers and thumbs. Push these over the knee cap and return down the sides of the knee area with the whole of the hands. Repeat four or five times, returning to the foot after the last stroke.

6. Repeat movement 2 three or four times.

A simple massage of the lower leg is given in detail in the Swiss Reflex Therapy chapter; this is useful when the whole leg does not need a massage.

## THE ABDOMEN

Massage of the abdomen is excellent for ensuring general well-being, relaxation and good digestion.

No pressure is ever applied with the thumbs or fingers in abdomen massage; any pressure is carried out with the palm

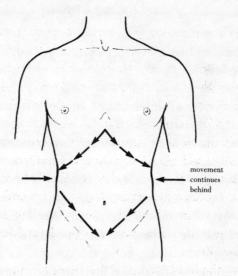

*Figure 33.* Movement 2 (abdomen).

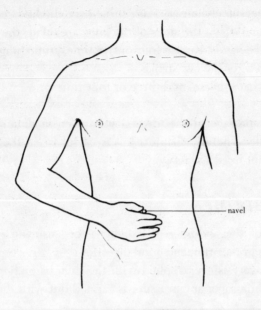

*Figure 34.* General Tension.

of the hand, and whenever pressure *is* applied, the recipient should be breathing out.

1.  Apply a small amount of oil all over the tummy and up to the rib cage.
2.  Place hands with overlapping fingers pointing towards the head exactly where the chest bone ends with the outside edges lying against (but not on) the rib cage. Pull the hands down and out toward the waist, turning the fingers so that they go under the body; pause; lift firmly upwards and pull the hands down and inwards (the outside edge lying against the hip bones this time) to the pelvic bone, returning lightly to the first position. Repeat this diamond shaped movement 3 or 4 times. (See Figure 33.)

3. Using the outside edge of both hands alternately, stroke down the left rib cage and then the right rib cage.

4. With reinforced palms of the hands do small circles in one big circle about 7½cm from the navel, slowly in a clockwise direction.

5. Place the palm of your hand over the centre of the abdomen, so that your thenar muscle (the big muscle of the thumb) is just touching the navel (see Figure 34). Place the palm of your other hand on top of the palm of the first hand and with gentle pressure do clockwise circles on the spot, not moving over the skin, but 'stuck to it' and moving the *skin* over the underlying tissue. Then, holding your hands still (in the same position), think healing thoughts about the person you are treating.

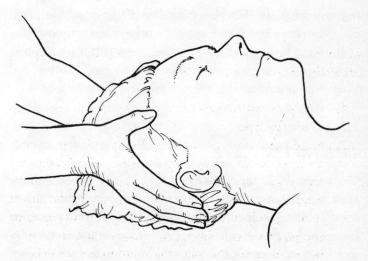

*Figure 35*. Movement 1 (scalp).

6. Effleurage up the centre of the tummy, round the rib cage and return down the sides of the body.
7. Repeat movement no. 2.

## THE SCALP

This is very relaxing for anyone who suffers from headaches and is best done with oil on your fingers from doing another part of the body. Oil put on the hands specially is lost on the hair itself.

1. Stand above the person's head and place the fingers all round the hairline as far as you can. Move up round the hairline then through the hair towards the top of the head to a comfortable position to draw your fingers out through the hair. Repeat five or six times. (See Figure 35.)
2. Hold all the fingers in contact with the scalp, as though stuck with glue and move the fingers *and* scalp over the bone beneath. (Do not move fingers through the hair *over* the scalp.) Change position and repeat. Change and repeat until all the scalp has had friction massage.
3. Repeat movement no. 1.

## THE FACE

The pressures in this massage are very good for headaches, eyestrain, sinuses and head colds. People with bronchitis or chest colds are helped tremendously by Swiss reflex therapy (see page 53) on the reflexes for sinuses, eyes and ears, spine, shoulders, neck and lungs, followed by aromatherapy massage using the right oils on the feet and legs, face and back. N.B. Numbers 3, 5 and 7 can be done on oneself for headaches,

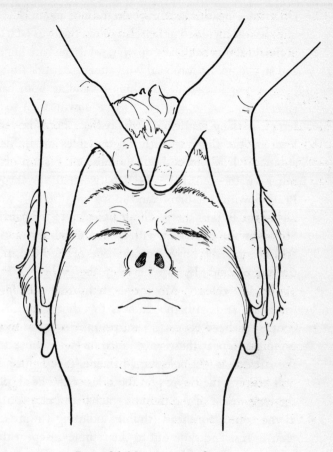

*Figure 36.* Movement 5 (face).

sinus or head colds to relieve congestion, but using your fingers, as this is easier.

1.   Put a very small amount of mixed oil into the palm of one hand. Rub both hands together and apply oil lightly all over the face, neck and upper chest.

2. Do gentle, upward effleurage on the face and neck, with both hands. Include light circles round the eyes (starting in the direction of the eyebrows), using the ring fingers, and stroke up the forehead with alternate hands (fingers lying across forehead), finishing by sliding both hands (turning fingers as you go, to face downwards) to the temples, where gentle but firm pressure should be given.

3. Keeping the fingers gently on the sides of the head, about ear level, place both thumbs one on top of the other on the centre forehead between the eyebrows. Press downwards firmly and move one thumb's width higher up. Repeat three or four times up to the hairline.

4. Stroke up the same area with alternate thumbs.

5. Still keeping the fingers on the side of the head, place the thumbs side by side between the eyebrows. Press firmly and release. Move one thumb's width *up* the forehead, and with the thumbs together again in the centre forehead repeat pressures, moving out towards temples. Repeat these rows once or twice more until the last one is just below the hairline. (See Figure 36.)

6. Still keeping the fingers on the sides of the head, place the big muscle of the thumbs (thenar muscle) to meet in the centre forehead (thumbs pointing towards the chin). Press and slide out to the temples. Repeat three or four times. (See Figure 37).

7. Leaving the thumbs on the forehead and using the second and third fingers, press and release on top of the cheekbone on the sides of the nose. Move one finger's width outwards, and press and release again. Repeat the pressures, following the crescent shape of the cheekbone, until almost at the temples. Move one finger's width *down* the crescent shape. If there is room, repeat again. (See Figure 38.)

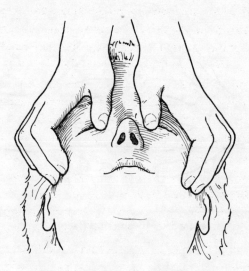

*Figure 37*. Movement 6 (face).

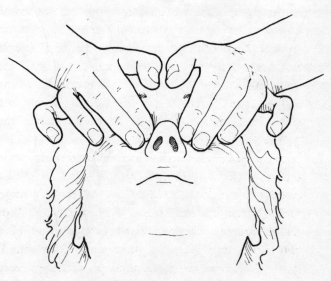

*Figure 38*. Movement 7 (face)

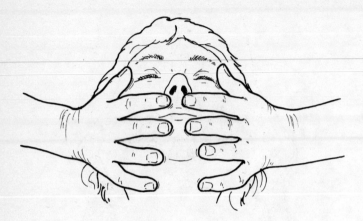

*Figure 39.* Movement 9 (face).

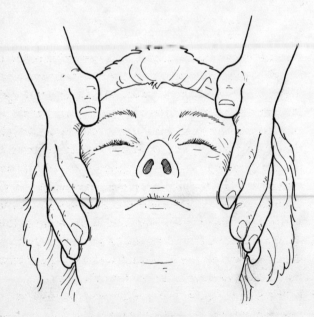

*Figure 40.* Movement 9 (face).

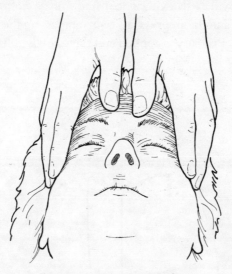

*Figure 41*. Movement 9 (face).

8. Return to the top of the nose, press and slide out to the temples with pressure, keeping the crescent shape. Move down one finger's width, and repeat; and again.

9*. Place the index fingers on the top lip, the middle and ring fingers below the lips (See Figure 39) and, hugging the face with the hand, pull out and up towards the temple (See Figure 40). Leave the fingers on the temple (Figure 41), lean back and place the thumb muscles onto the centre of the forehead, and slide with pressure to meet the fingers, which are still at the temples (look again at Figure 37). Lift up the fingers and, leaving the thenar muscle on the temples, lean forward and repeat the whole movement three or four times more.

10. Follow Figure 42 for the facial pressure points – in each case use the ring or middle fingers. The fingers should

(and will with experience) find a little hollow to slip into, and then press at right angles to the pressure point. Pressure is applied and then slowly released.

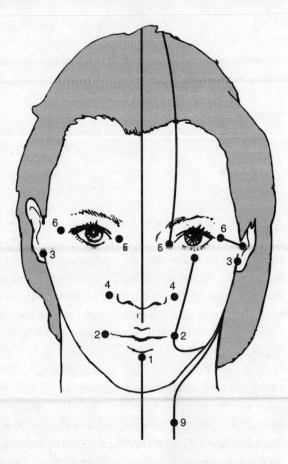

*Figure 42.* Pressure points of the face.

a. between the lower lip and chin (press with one finger on top of the other)

b. just beyond the mouth corners

c. about 2½cm in front of the ear lobe base, just below the jaw bone

d. on either side of the nostrils; feel for a little hollow just below the cheek bones

e. just above the inside corner of the eye, on the bone; press upwards

f. about 2½cm from the outside corner of the eye right on the temples, feel until a little hollow is found.

11. Repeat movement no.2, including this time effleurage from the top of the neck down to and across the chest, round the shoulder blades and back to the top of the neck. Finish with eye and forehead stroking, this time making the alternate forehead strokes slower and slower, until you no longer put the second hand onto the head, but just bring the other very slowly off, the little finger being the last thing to leave the forehead.

## THE ARMS

These can be best done in a sitting position.

1. Spread the oil over the arms in the usual way, and (holding the hand with one hand) do effleurage strokes over the whole arm with the other. Change hands and do the inside arm.

2. Friction movements can be done where there are problem areas, e.g., rheumatism or arthritis, adapting whatever is suitable from movements already learnt.

3. Stroke up the centre of the palm with the thumbs (supporting the hand with the fingers behind) over the thenar* muscle and outer side of the hand.
4. Do zig-zag movements down the palm with the whole of the thumbs and push firmly back up towards wrist.
5. Do zig-zag movements on both sides of the wrist.
6. Effleurage on the back of the hand with the whole of the thumbs.
7. Repeat effleurage in movement no. 1.

* Big thumb muscle on side of palm.

## THE SHOULDERS

Quite often there is tension in the upper neck and shoulder area, extending to the base of the shoulder blade. This is sometimes easier to treat in a sitting position where you can get right on top of the shoulder itself and do kneading or petrissage there.

1. Apply oil in the usual way and do soothing effleurage strokes around the shoulder blades.
2. Using the thumbs, do alternate strokes just to the left hand side of the spine up to the neck and up to the neck itself to the hairline if necessary.
3. Pick up, squeeze and release the top shoulder muscle from the shoulder edge along the neck.
4. Do alternate strokes with thumbs up top of shoulder towards neck and up neck if necessary.
5. Using thumbs again do friction massage over any nodules in the shoulders themselves.
6. Repeat the effleurage in No. 1.

## LOWER LEG MASSAGE

The following massage is useful for those who suffer from cramp in their calves or feet and can also be done after a Swiss reflex treatment or simply for its own merits.

1.  Apply a small amount of oil all over one leg (with the other leg wrapped in a towel to keep it warm).
2.  Effleurage up the front of the leg, using both hands with fingers facing one another and gently return down sides. Repeat 3 times.
3.  Effleurage up the back of the leg and return down sides 3 times.
4.  Effleurage firmly up the back of the leg, taking calf muscle to the side and returning to the ankle. Repeat 4 times.
5.  Repeat, using the other hand and taking muscle to the other side.
6.  Repeat, using each hand alternately and working a little further down the leg with each stroke, finishing on Achilles tendon.
7.  Do numbers 4, 6 and 7 from the foot massage.
8.  Repeat number 2.

*chapter nine*

## PREPARING OILS
## FOR MASSAGE

We have to have some medium with which we carry out massage movements – something to help our hands to move over the skin evenly. Some masseurs use talcum powder, but this can be very drying; most use some form of vegetable or mineral oil. For the massage movements alone to be effective, any of the three mediums can be used. But for aromatherapy it is necessary to choose something which will 'carry' the chosen essential oils (which themselves are not, despite their name, oily or greasy) through the skin and into the blood circulation ... so we have to use oil rather than powder.

Mineral oil is useless, because although essential oils will dissolve in it, it has a very low penetration power (hence its use as baby oil) so the essential oil is restricted in its attempt to pass through the skin. Certain less viscous vegetable oils are ideal, as they are of themselves fairly penetrative and therefore do not hinder the highly penetrative essential oils from getting into the blood stream. It is preferable that a good quality vegetable oil is chosen as a carrier to hasten the curative effects of the essential oils you put in it. Only just enough is needed to be able to move smoothly over the area being massaged. If too much is used, you will slip or slide over the area, wasting the oil and not doing much good with your movements.

There are several good vegetable oil bases which can be used for blending. The choice is usually dependent on any health giving properties the oil may have, but it may also, (for some people) be dependent on the smell and texture of the oil.

All carrier oils must of course be 100 per cent pure unrefined oils for maximum penetration (cold pressed where possible), and usually the higher the price the more genuine the oil.

Avocado and hazlenut oils possibly penetrate the skin the most easily; avocado and wheat germ oils are the most nourishing. Calendula and hypericum are rather special carrier oils (explained in greater detail on page 117), they are both anti-inflammatory and therefore useful on bruises and sprains. Other properties they possess are on page 117. Grapeseed, olive, peachnut, sweet almond, corn, soya bean and sunflower seed oils are all good basic oils, not varying a great deal in effect, but varying in aroma (very important), penetration, price (quite a lot), and keeping qualities (also very important).

Grapeseed is the only one of the above oils which is never cold pressed. It is possible to rescue the oil before it is completely refined, which increases the cost somewhat but gives a better oil for aromatherapy. As more becomes known about the effects of certain cold pressed carrier oils on the skin, the more important becomes the choice of carrier oil to be used with your essential oils. For example:

- sunflower is helpful for inflamed joints and bruises,
- hazlenut is useful on an oily skin – and has a sun factor of 10, according to research done in Chile,
- rosehip is regenerative, being effective on wounds, scars, eczema and ageing
- evening primrose is beneficial to eczema and psoriasis,
- jojoba (which is a liquid wax) is helpful for rheumatism,

acne and sunburnt skin – as well as for eczema and psoriasis.

Any of these oils can be used on their own, or blended with vegetable oil, but if a bottle of massage oil is being made up for daily use, then 5–10 per cent of wheatgerm oil (which is anti-oxidant), should be added to help the keeping qualities; corn oil is not a good choice, as its keeping qualities are the least good. Vegetable oils tend to oxidize and turn rancid much more quickly than essential oils, so be careful to store in a dark, cool cupboard. When adding essential oils never mix more than a couple of months supply (50–100ml) at any one time, and always add 5 per cent of wheatgerm oil to the mix.

Wheatgerm oil is also good for a dry skin, and the percentage used can be increased if wished, but it is rarely used on its own as it is too rich, too heavy and also more expensive!

Avocado is another rich, heavier and more expensive carrier oil which is rarely used on its own. It, too, is good for a dry skin, and it is usually added to grapeseed (or other base oil) to help penetration, as its penetrative powers (along with hazelnut oil) are greater than other carrier oils. So 5–10 per cent can be added to the mix for speedier penetration or if the person being massaged has a lot of fatty tissue.

Thus it is possible for a 50ml bottle of carrier oil to be made up as follows:

1 teaspoonful wheatgerm oil
1 teaspoonful avocado or hazelnut oil
Fill up with basic carrier oil or oils          } into bottle
(the choice depending on the extra
benefit the carrier oil or oils can give
to your problem)

It is then ready to add the therapeutic element: the essential oils.

Some therapeutic plants – such as calendula – contain so little essential oil that it is too expensive to distil them. Instead, such plants can be macerated in one of the base carrier oils, usually olive or sunflower. The chopped-up plant material is put in a giant mixer with the base oil and turned with the blades for several days, after which the plant has released any therapeutic constituents which are soluble in the vegetable oil and is ready to filter before bottling. Oils obtained this way, by maceration, are:

* calendula, a well known skin healer (properties below)
* carrot (from the roots; the seeds produce an essential oil), anti-inflammatory and rejuvenating
* hypericum (St John's Wort) also well known, anti-inflammatory and useful on bruises
* lime blossom, rejuvenating and relaxing
* melissa (whose leaves are also distilled to produce an essential oil), beneficial on mature, dry skin and fluid retention (as is also melissa water).

Calendula (*Calendula officinalis*, often referred to as marigold) is possibly the best known macerated oil, and is not to be confused with the marigold essential oil from *Tagetes glandulifera*, which is from the same family. Calendula is of Egyptian origin and is valued there as a medicinal plant. The petals of the plant contain carotene and can be used in salads or cooked with rice to colour it yellow instead of saffron. Calendula oil is quite expensive so aromatherapists often use it with another carrier oil plus the essential oils. Calendula is anti-inflammatory and excellent for disorders such as:

* chillblains and rheumatic joints

- skin problems – such as eczema and chapped and cracked skin
- broken and varicose veins
- burns, wounds and ulcers
- sprains and bruises

Another popular macerated carrier oil is hypericum. It is also known as St John's Wort, possibly because the flowers are at their best for macerating in July, when St John was beheaded – and because the yellow buds, when squeezed, release hypericin (responsible for the plant's healing powers) which is a blood red liquid and stains the fingers.

Hypericum is also anti-inflammatory (and slightly analgesic); it is helpful for:

- sprains, bruises and burns (including sunburn)
- rheumatism
- haemorrhoids
- wounds

## ESSENTIAL OILS AND CARRIERS

It is important to select the correct quantity of essential oil to put into the carrier oil. This depends to a large extent on the area to be covered during any one treatment. Aromatherapy, as carried out by complementary therapists is a *total* treatment, and is usually carried out on the face, scalp, body, legs and arms. When you are helping a particular ailment yourself, such as arthritis, you need only do the part of the body giving the problem.

For some ailments though (and for some people), using a carrier *oil* is not always practical. It is possible to use very successfully a carrier *lotion* instead. I have mine made up for me and it is completely vegetable based and non-greasy.

For anyone interested in this lotion write to Shirley Price Aromatherapy (for address see page 220).

It is worth mentioning here that many essential oils have normalizing effects; i.e., they will sedate or uplift, relax or stimulate, and will successfully treat an oily or a dry skin. The result obtained depends on the condition of the person being treated.

A minute proportion of the chosen oils can effect a cure, as in the case of digitalis extract mentioned earlier. Usually, the more toxic the essence the smaller should be the quantity used. Sage and fennel are relatively more toxic than most oils. Rose, lavender and chamomile have a very low toxicity. None of the essential oils on our retail list is toxic when used correctly, as advised.

Some problems respond better to a very dilute essential oil, while others, requiring the same oil to be used for the treatment, may need a greater strength to respond positively. It will be found that trial and error sometimes play a very big part in determining the concentration of oil to use for a particular person for a specific complaint.

This is confusing to the beginner but expertise and confidence will soon be acquired by experience. It is best initially to use the average percentage given or less, and only if this does not give the desired result should the concentration be increased. It does not necessarily follow that the more you use the better will be the effect – in fact it is often the reverse.

Lower concentrations often give as good or better results if the problem is emotional, but if you are working mainly on a physical problem then a higher concentration would probably produce better results.

*Chapter ten*

# RECIPES

The table on pages 138–181 gives a description of many of the essential oils available, with a list of their uses. The most popular, useful and interesting oils have been included. The list is in three sections: top note oils, which are mainly stimulating and uplifting; middle note oils, which cover most bodily ailments; and base note oils, which are mainly sedative.

The most useful reference list, however, is the therapeutic index of selected problems on page 182 and it will be found invaluable for information concerning the oils to treat a specific condition.

Therapeutically, most of the problems one comes up against can be dealt with by the less expensive oils (lavender is particularly useful), but neroli (orange flower) and rose otto are unbeatable for their delightful aromas and excellent effects on complaints of nervous origin, e.g., tension, anxiety and stress. Jasmine, orange blossom and rose absolutes can also be helpful, but remember these are not essential oils and if a poor quality, may cause a skin reaction due to any remaining solvent or added adulterant.

Genuine essential oils can be used in several ways – to make a tea, to use in the bath, to mix in a massage oil, etc. If you want to use the essential oils in all these ways it is beneficial to use a 10ml dropper bottle and mix, say, 20 drops each of the oils you have chosen for your condition (let us assume muscle cramp) so that you have a ready mixed treatment bottle (which you can label 'cramp') of pure essential oils from which you can make your tea, add to carrier oils for massage, or put in the bath, etc.

And now we come to the exciting part! Selecting which oils to use!

You will find when you turn to the therapeutic index not only that several oils will treat one symptom, but also that one oil will treat several symptoms, so first of all write down the condition you are wanting to treat the most, e.g., you may be suffering from rheumatism and migraine. Decide which condition gives you the most discomfort. Let us suppose it is the migraine. Now write down all the essential oils which will help migraine (see the therapeutic index).

'migraine: eucalyptus, Roman chamomile, lavender, lemon, marjoram (sweet), melissa, peppermint, rosemary, rose otto'

Well, we can't use all of those! If you suffer from migraine alone, then choose from the above oils any two to four oils (never more than four) to get the right aroma for you. But as we want to treat your rheumatism as well if we can, turn to 'rheumatism' and see if any of the oils for migraine repeat themselves.

'rheumatism: *eucalyptus*, lemon, sage, thyme, *Roman chamomile*, juniper, hyssop, *lavender, marjoram (sweet), rosemary*'

So eucalyptus, Roman chamomile, lavender, sweet marjoram and rosemary will treat both your rheumatism *and* your migraine.

First of all, put one drop each of any two or three of these oils into a teaspoonful of carrier oil (in an egg cup), mix and rub a little onto the back of your hand. Does it smell nice? If you like it, those are the oils to use. If you have used eucalyptus or Roman chamomile and they are too predominant, put in one extra drop of either lavender, sweet marjoram or rosemary, whichever aroma you prefer, or even one drop of rose otto if you think it would make it smell nicer for your personal preference, because this will be an additional help to your migraine, which is your first concern.

Another example; let us suppose now that tension is largely responsible for your condition, which in this case is migraine and irregular periods. So we write down all the oils for tension.

'tension: basil, bergamot, Roman chamomile, lavender, frankincense, geranium, marjoram, melissa, neroli, rose otto and ylang-ylang'

What a long list! If it is only tension you want to treat, then use any two to three of these oils to make the most relaxing aroma for you. Remember top notes have a sharper aroma, middle notes vary a great deal but are never woody or heavy, base notes are much sweeter and heavier; so decide whether you like a light or a heavy aroma and choose accordingly. We want to treat migraine as well, so write down the oils for that condition which already appear on the tension list, e.g.,

'migraine: *Roman chamomile, lavender, sweet marjoram, melissa and rose otto*'

If you now turn to irregular periods you will find that Roman chamomile, lavender, melissa and rose otto are the oils mentioned there. As these four oils occur in each ailment, they are the best oils to use for treatment. When the oils match up as well as this, use equal drops of each in your mix. However, occasionally, you will find that the oils don't always match up as easily as these examples. If not, don't worry; just make sure you put in more drops of the oil which helps the most important problem. For example, if you needed 8 drops in total, and have two problems for which the oils don't match up well, use 5 drops of the one indicated for the first problem and 3 for the second. Similarly, if you want to help three problems and you find that all the oils are different, just adjust the number of drops of the main oil you need. Used in synergy like this (i.e. using more than one essential oil) you will find that each oil has a more powerful effect – and even the problem for which you used the least number of drops will benefit.

It is a fascinating occupation choosing and mixing essential oils for use in aromatherapy, and with experience the most effective blend for your particular problem can be worked out. Meanwhile, I will help you with suggested 'recipes' to start you off, and also tell you which oils blend well together for a particular complaint. For pure aroma, on the Table of Essential Oils (see pages 133–181) you will find a list of some other oils with which each blends best. As you know from buying or being given perfumes, certain 'smells' suit some people and not others, so I can only suggest what is acceptable to me. You must find your own end aroma, and the best way of doing that is by trying different combinations of the selected treatment oils.

Any oil can of course be used on its own. In the last example, melissa, rose otto *or* Roman chamomile could be tried if the aroma is pleasing.

For some conditions you will find that it can be difficult to arrive at a totally acceptable aroma. So then add a drop or two

of any oil which you feel will make the treatment oil acceptable. Geranium, lemon, sweet orange and sandalwood are of
particular use here.

No essential oil is 'nice' to take internally, except in tea. Tea
to which essential oils are added has to be very weak and one
can learn to accept the flavour if it means good health, but as
there will be at least a thousand combinations, even if you
only possess a small selection of oils it should be possible to
arrive at a flavour you can enjoy.

Never forget the importance of the attitude of mind in ill-
health. Illness is not always completely physical (see Chapter
1). Remember too, that a small percentage of oil will usually
treat a psychological condition whereas a stronger percentage
is usually required for a purely physical complaint.

When mixing essential oils together (neat, for one condition, to be used in a variety of ways), a hypodermic syringe
(usually obtainable from your local chemist) is an ideal way of
measuring the quantities, and much quicker than counting a
lot of drops. But don't forget to put a label on the bottle (with
the date), and write on it what you have used, for example,

| *Indigestion* | | *Indigestion* |
|---|---|---|
| 2ml peppermint | | 40 drops peppermint |
| 1ml chamomile | or | 20 drops chamomile |
| 1ml fennel | | 20 drops fennel |

Before giving you the recipes which I have tried (and had success with) on clients, may I remind you that as I said earlier
not everyone reacts in the same way to a certain blend, and I
have often had to choose an alternative blend for someone
where the first did not have the desired effect.

All the recipes are given in numbers which can be used
either as drops or millilitres; this means that you can mix a

small amount of essential oils in drops – just to try it out – and see if the mix is a successful one for your problem. (N.B. to mix a small amount for application or massage, use only one drop of each oil mentioned – two where there are double figures – in two teaspoonsful of carrier oil.) When you find a recipe that suits you, you can then use the numbers to mix a larger amount of essential oils in millilitres (with your syringe), into a small bottle with a dropper. This will save a lot of time and trouble, giving you a ready mixed quantity for use in several ways; in a bath or a compress, for application, inhalation or in a tea (for the latter, never put essential oils directly into a cup of tea – always make a *pot*).

| | |
|---|---|
| Baths | 6–8 drops (also foot and hand baths) |
| Compress | 2–8 drops in ½ cup of water (100ml) |
| Ingestion | 2–3 drops in red wine or honey and water 2–3 times daily (see Author's Note at the beginning of the book) |
| Inhalant | 6–10 drops on paper towel 3–5 drops in ½ basin hot water |
| Massage Oil | 15–30 drops in 50ml carrier oil |
| Tea | 2–3 drops on one tea bag for 3–4 cups of tea, without milk. Drink one cup 3 times daily |

The number of drops recommended above for each method of use are averages; the amount any individual may need can vary – and an exact number is not crucial to the success of the treatment. You will see in the table that I have (for physical problems) given a larger number of drops than the average normally used in the bath or for massage; this is because I found these quantities more successful for the needs of the particular client I was treating.

Throughout the table, 'App/Mass' is short for applying to yourself (self-application) or using for massage. For massage, always use a carrier oil (basic, macerated or a blend of two or morc. For self-application, an oil *can* be used, but it is difficult to estimate the correct quantity to use on a small area – and can result in clothes being spoilt by the oil. It is much easier to use a carrier lotion, which is easier to handle and disappears into the skin, leaving it satin smooth and not at all oily. If you need the benefits of one of the macerated (or basic) vegetable oils, you can always add up to 20 per cent into your lotion (a little at a time) – and it will still not be greasy.

Remember you can *decrease* the dose for psychological problems and *increase* it for physical problems, but at no time use more than 10 drops for any *one* treatment; you may hinder the beneficial effect. You may of course use more than one treatment technique in any one day e.g. drink tea, put oils in the bath and use a compress or massage oil.

For the methods of using essential oils in the following recipes turn to the chapters on Simple Aromatherapy Treatment Techniques and Aromatherapy Massage Techniques.

If you would find it more convenient to have oils ready mixed, these can be obtained from the address at the back of this book.

## Anti-stretch Marks

|  | Frankincense | Lavender | Lemongrass |
|---|---|---|---|
| Massage Oil (not lotion) | 10 | 15 | 5 |

## Arthritis (& Joints)

|  | Benzoin* | Chamomile | Rosemary | Lavandin |
|---|---|---|---|---|
| Bath | 2 | 1 | 2 | 3 |
| App/Mass | 6 | 6 | 8 | 8 |
| Tea | — | 1 | 1 | |

|  | Lavender | Rosemary | Marjoram |
|---|---|---|---|
| Bath | 2 | 2 | 3 |
| App/Mass | 8 | 8 | 12 |
| Tea | — | — | 2 |

## Arthritis and Rheumatism

|  | Eucalyptus | Juniper | Marjoram | Rosemary |
|---|---|---|---|---|
| Bath | 1 | 2 | 2 | 3 |
| App/Mass | 6 | 8 | 6 | 8 |
| Tea | — | — | 1 | 1 |

## Bronchitis

|  | Eucalyptus | Niaouli | Sandalwood |
|---|---|---|---|
| Bath | 4 | 2 | 2 |
| Compress | 6 | 2 | 2 |
| Inhalant | 6 | 2 | 2 |
| App/Mass | 15 | 5 | 5 |

\* Resins and absolutes should not be used in acrylic baths unless diluted first.

### Cellulite (& Hangover!)

|          | Fennel | Juniper | Rosemary |
|----------|--------|---------|----------|
| Bath     | 4      | 1       | 2        |
| App/Mass | 12     | 4       | 8        |

### Chilblains

|          | Lemon | Cypress | Lavender |
|----------|-------|---------|----------|
| Compress | 3     | 3       | 3        |
| App/Mass | 15    | 5       | 5        |

### Cold in the Head

|          | Basil | Eucalyptus | Peppermint |
|----------|-------|------------|------------|
| Bath     | 3     | 3          | 2          |
| Inhalant | 3     | 3          | 2          |

### Cough & Cold

|          | Lemon | Bl. Pepper | Eucalyptus | Sandalwood |
|----------|-------|------------|------------|------------|
| Bath     | —     | 3          | 3          | 2          |
| Inhalant | 2     | 1          | 2          | 2          |

### Cramp

|          | Basil | Marjoram |
|----------|-------|----------|
| Bath     | 4     | 4        |
| App/Mass | 15    | 15       |

|          | Basil | Cypress | Marjoram |
|----------|-------|---------|----------|
| Bath     | 4     | 2       | 2        |
| App/Mass | 12    | 8       | 8        |

### Dermatitis

|            | Geranium | Juniper | Lavender |
|------------|----------|---------|----------|
| Bath       | 4        | 2       | 2        |
| App/Mass   | 12       | 6       | 6        |

### Eczema

|             | Bergamot | Geranium | Juniper | Lavender |
|-------------|----------|----------|---------|----------|
| Compress    | 2        | 2        | 2       | 2        |
| Massage Oil | 5        | 5        | 5       | 5        |

### High Blood Pressure

|          | Lavender | Ylang-ylang | Lemon |
|----------|----------|-------------|-------|
| Bath     | 5        | 3           | 2     |
| App/Mass | 10       | 10          | 10    |
| Tea      | 0        | 1           | 1     |

### Indigestion

|          | Mandarin | Bergamot | Peppermint |
|----------|----------|----------|------------|
| App/Mass | 6        | 6        | 12         |
| Tea      | 1        | 1        | 1          |

|          | Fennel | Peppermint | Bl. Pepper |
|----------|--------|------------|------------|
| App/Mass | 6      | 6          | 6          |
| Tea      | 1      | 1          | 1          |

### Insect Repellent

|          | Eucalyptus | Peppermint | Cedarwood |
|----------|------------|------------|-----------|
| App/Mass | 12         | 6          | 6         |

### Insomnia

|      | Chamomile | Juniper | Marjoram | Rose Otto |
|------|-----------|---------|----------|-----------|
| Bath | 2         | 2       | 3        | 1         |
| Tea  | 1         | 1       | —        | —         |

### Insomnia & Stress

|      | Chamomile | Juniper | Marjoram |
|------|-----------|---------|----------|
| Bath | 2         | 4       | 2        |
| Tea  | 1         | —       | 1        |

|         | Chamomile | Juniper | Neroli |
|---------|-----------|---------|--------|
| Bath    | 2         | 2       | 4      |
| Tea (1) | —         | —       | 2      |
| Tea (2) | 1         | —       | 1      |

### Irregular Periods

|          | Chamomile | Melissa | Rose Otto |
|----------|-----------|---------|-----------|
| Bath     | 2         | 3       | 3         |
| Compress | 4         | 4       | 4         |
| App/Mass | 6         | 10      | 10        |

### Migraine & Rheumatism

|          | Lavender | Marjoram | Rosemary | Chamomile |
|----------|----------|----------|----------|-----------|
| Bath     | 2        | 2        | 2        | 2         |
| Compress | 2        | 2        | 4        | 2         |
| App/Mass | 5        | 5        | 10       | 10        |
| Tea      | 1        | 1        | 1        | —         |

### Muscular Aches & Pains

|                | Eucalyptus | Rosemary | Lavandin |
|----------------|------------|----------|----------|
| Bath           | 2          | 3        | 3        |
| Compress       | 3          | 3        | 4        |
| Hand/Foot Bath | 3          | 3        | 4        |
| App/Mass       | 8          | 8        | 12       |

### Muscle Tone

|          | Bl. Pepper | Lavender | Lemon |
|----------|------------|----------|-------|
| Bath     | 3          | 2        | 3     |
| App/Mass | 12         | 8        | 8     |

### Nervous Tension

|              | Bergamot | Marjoram | Neroli | Sandalwood |
| ------------ | -------- | -------- | ------ | ---------- |
| Bath (1)     | —        | —        | 5      | 1          |
| Bath (2)     | 2        | 2        | 1      | 2          |
| Massage Oil  | 4        | 4        | 4      | 4          |
| Tea (1)      | 1        | —        | —      | 1          |
| Tea (2)      | —        | —        | 2      | —          |

### Nervous Tension

|              | Basil | Juniper | Lavender | Ylang-ylang |
| ------------ | ----- | ------- | -------- | ----------- |
| Bath         | 1     | 2       | 2        | 1           |
| App/Mass (1) | 4     | 4       | 4        | 4           |
| App/Mass (2) | —     | —       | 6        | 12          |
| Tea          | —     | —       | 1        | 1           |

### Perspiring Feet

|           | Bergamot | Clary-sage | Cypress |
| --------- | -------- | ---------- | ------- |
| Foot Bath | 4        | 4          | 2       |

### Poor Circulation

|          | Benzoin | Bl. Pepper | Juniper |
| -------- | ------- | ---------- | ------- |
| Bath     | —       | 4          | 4       |
| App/Mass | 8       | 12         | 12      |
| Tea      | —       | 1          | 1       |

### Sinus Problems

|          | Basil | Eucalyptus | Lavender | Peppermint |
| -------- | ----- | ---------- | -------- | ---------- |
| Bath     | 2     | 2          | 2        | 2          |
| Inhalant | 2     | 2          | 2        | 2          |
| App/Mass | 5     | 5          | 5        | 5          |

### Tonic for Hair

| Cedarwood | Juniper | Rosemary |
|:---------:|:-------:|:--------:|
| 10 | 10 | 15 |

Use in 50ml surgical spirit (or flower water if hair very greasy), not carrier oil or lotion.

*Chapter eleven*

◑⟩⟩

# TABLE OF ESSENTIAL OILS

## *HOW PURE IS AN ESSENTIAL OIL?*

This is not an easy question to answer, because industrial production is not necessarily a simple procedure. We have already
seen in Chapter 2 that only distilled and expressed oils are
pure enough to be called essential oils, but even these are
open to adulteration, or sometimes, to 'blending'.

**Adulteration** of an essential oil can be done at various
stages, though rarely from a small distillation source; it is usually the large commercial distillers who deal in hundreds of
tonnes who 'stretch', 'ennoble' or otherwise adulterate their
oils. Companies interested in natural or organic growing (for
medicinal use) have their plants distilled in newer, smaller,
stainless steel stills – the quantities grown are much less than
the hundreds of acres of plants grown for the huge demands
of the perfume and food industries.

Because of the soil variation and the weather, the components of an essential oil may vary slightly in percentage
present at each harvest. This does not affect its therapeutic
value, but can affect the aroma, which is what the food and
perfume industries are interested in. Adulteration (either with
components taken from another essential oil, or synthetic

substitutes) is the only way for these two industries to ensure that they have oils with exactly the same composition each time they need a new supply. Adulterated oils are much less expensive than the genuine article, but if used for therapeutics, the quantity needed to have a beneficial effect on the health may be greater. There may also be a risk of side effects due to an added synthetic component or to something which has come from a herbicide or pesticide used in the growing (these have molecules which are small enough to be distilled) and are therefore in the oil itself. For guaranteed beneficial results, oils which are grown without pesticides and herbicides, or have a certificate for organic growth, should always be obtained.

A '**blend**' can be many different things:

- a mix of essential oils, undiluted, of good quality and selected for their combined therapeutic effects
- a mix of essential oils in a vegetable oil (whatever the quantity) ready to apply to the skin
- a mix of essential oils, adulterated in some way (therefore of poor quality) and sold as an oil from a single plant, for example:

    a) rosemary oil which has had camphor (which is very cheap) or a synthetic component added to it to make it less expensive.
    b) 'melissa' oil made by blending together several cheap citral-type essential oils (with or without added synthetic components) to give an aroma near to that of melissa. Such melissa oil is very cheap to buy, unlike genuine melissa, which is very expensive – at least 10 times the price!

So you can see that commercially blended oils, which are quite suitable for the perfumery trade, do not have the correct therapeutic attributes we need for aromatherapy, and therefore cannot be classed as pure essential oils by an aromatherapist.

Being natural products, the quantity, quality and therefore the properties of essential oils vary from season to season with weather conditions, etc., as I have already said earlier in the book, so the price varies accordingly with each harvest. Price also varies with the amount of oil found in a plant; for example, eucalyptus leaves are rich in oil but jasmine and rose petals, melissa leaves and orange flowers contain only a little. Therefore you must expect to pay up from six to *twelve* times as much for these four oils as for most other oils, because much larger quantities of petals (or leaves in the case of melissa) are required to yield a given amount of oil, and much more work is involved. It is possible to buy in stores and some herbal shops jasmine and other oils which are diluted in some form, either with alcohol or carrier oil. The label may not state that it has been diluted, but the price should tell you! This means you could use it as a 'ready mixed' oil (if it is diluted in vegetable oil) but it could not be used in the recipes given in this book, all of which require undiluted, unblended pure essential oils.

Selecting an essential oil for therapeutic use is full of traps for the unwary or inexperienced, and the wisest course of action is to obtain supplies only from an honest, reliable source in whom you can trust. This element of trust is most important in the essential oil business, as the selection of pure oils is very much an art, combined with knowledge and wide experience.

## *TABLE OF ESSENTIAL OILS*

### *Alphabetical List of Oils*

| Name | Note | General Effect |
| --- | --- | --- |
| Aniseed | Middle | Warming and stimulating |
| Basil | Top | Uplifting and refreshing |
| Benzoin | Base | Warming and relaxing |
| Bergamot | Top | Uplifting and refreshing; also relaxing |
| Black Pepper | Middle | Stimulating |
| Cajuput | Top | Antiseptic and warming |
| Chamomile | Middle | Refreshing and relaxing |
| Caraway | Top to Middle | Warming and stimulating |
| Cedarwood | Base | Sedative |
| Clary-sage | Top to Middle | Warming and relaxing |
| Clove | Base to Middle | Antiseptic and warming |
| Coriander | Top to Middle | Warming and stimulating |
| Cypress | Middle to Base | Relaxing and refreshing |
| Eucalyptus | Top | Head clearing |
| Fennel | Middle | Carminative (eases wind and stomach pains) |
| Frankincense | Base | Relaxing and rejuvenating |
| Geranium | Middle | Refreshing and relaxing |
| Ginger | Base | Warming and digestive |
| Hyssop | Middle | Decongestant (respiratory) |
| Jasmine | Base | Relaxing and soothing |
| Juniper | Middle | Refreshing, stimulating and relaxing |
| Lavender | Middle | Refreshing, relaxing, generally therapeutic |
| Lemon | Top | Refreshing and stimulating |
| Lemongrass | Top | Toning and refreshing |
| Marjoram | Middle | Warming and fortifying |

| Melissa | Middle | Uplifting and refreshing |
| Myrrh | Base | Cooling and toning |
| Neroli | Base to Middle | Ultra-relaxing |
| Niaouli | Top | Antiseptic and analgesic |
| Nutmeg | Base to Middle | Warming and digestive |
| Orange | Top | Refreshing, relaxing |
| Origanum | Base | Antiseptic, sedative, warming |
| Patchouli | Base | Relaxing |
| Peppermint | Middle to Top | Cooling and refreshing |
| Petitgrain | Top | Refreshing and relaxing |
| Pine Needle | Middle to Base | Refreshing and antiseptic |
| Rose Otto | Base to Middle | Relaxing and soothing |
| Rosemary | Middle | Invigorating and refreshing |
| Sage | Top | Decongestant (circulatory) |
| Sandalwood | Base | Relaxing |
| Savory | Middle | Stimulating and warming |
| Tea Tree | Top | Excellent antiseptic |
| Thyme | Top to Middle | Antiseptic |
| Ylang-Ylang | Base | Relaxing |

Whether or not an oil is classed as top, middle or base is very subjective. The only way really to test this is by dipping a spill into an oil and leaving it in a room of normal temperature.

**top notes** – the aroma lasts up to 24 hours.
**middle notes** – the aroma lasts two to three days.
**base notes** – the aroma is still there after one week.

The fact that essential oils have an aromatic 'life span' is much more important to a perfumer than to an aromatherapist, whose aims are for penetration into the body, rather than the length of time it will last on the skin surface before losing its strength.

It should also be remembered that when essential oils are blended together their aromatic life span is altered, depending on the mixture. This fact, too, is of more importance to the perfumer, though sometimes helpful to the aromatherapist.

In the following table my own suggestions for blending are given. Lavender usually blends well with any oil; after that it is much a question of personal preference, as in the choice of a perfume. If an aroma is desired solely as a perfume, up to 12 or 15 oils can be used to obtain an individual aroma; however, for therapeutic use it is generally recognized that 5 is the maximum, 3–4 being preferred.

## TOP NOTES

These are all stimulating and uplifting.

**Basil** *(Ocimum basilicum* var. *album)*

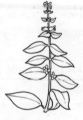

*Blends well with:*
bergamot
geranium
lavender

There are many varieties of sweet basil, which belongs to the Lamiaceae family. It originated in Asia and was extensively used in Indian medicine. More often grown now in Reunion, France, Cyprus and the Seychelles. The flowering tops and leaves are used and extraction is by distillation. The leaves are supposed to be a love symbol in Italy. It is an oil which clears the head and is uplifting – it makes a good nerve tonic.

Circulation: low blood pressure

Digestive: indigestion, intestinal infections, gastro-enteritis, flatulence, sluggish digestion, travel sickness

Head: earache, colds, migraine, vertigo (dizziness)

Muscular: spasm (cramp), rheumatoid arthritis

Menstrual: uterine congestion

Nervous: anxiety, depression, mental strain, nervous debility, tonic, nervous insomnia

Skin: dry eczema, sluggish or congested, insect repellent, soothes wasp stings (use neat)

Special: gout

*Note:* Basil oils containing a high percentage of methyl chavicol should be used with care.

**Bergamot** *(Citrus bergamia)*

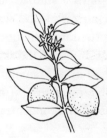

*Blends well with:*
cypress
jasmine
lavender
neroli

Bergamot belongs to the Rutaceae family. The oil is obtained by expression from the fresh peel of the fruit after the juice has been extracted. The main production area is southern Italy. The trees grow to a height of 15 feet (4.5m), and fruits are picked December to February. The fruits, which are somewhere between an orange and a lemon in shape, change from green to yellow and the newly ripe fruits give the best oil.

The oil yield is half a kilo from 100 kilos of fruit and the colour is yellowish to browny green. The essential oil is used in the production of Earl Grey tea. Bergamot oil is liable to skilful adulteration and is used prominently in eau-de-cologne and lavender water.

It is a powerful antiseptic and is helpful when used in the bath in the case of vaginal pruritis. It is excellent (personal experience) against cold sores, especially when the first tender signs become apparent (see *Note* below).

Digestive: colic, flatulence, indigestion, loss of appetite, stomach pains, tonic
Head: sore throat, tonsillitis
Nervous: agitation, anxiety, depression
Skin: herpes simplex I (cold sore), psoriasis, eczema

*Note:* Do not apply to a cold sore just before going into the sun (or onto a sunbed) as pigmentation will occur on the site of contact; always wait 2 or 3 hours, to give it time to be absorbed into the body. Because bergamot increases the photosensitivity of the skin, it was once used in sun preparations, to hasten the tanning process. However, because there were problems with it (many people were burned), it is now banned in a concentration of more than 0.001 per cent.

**Cajuput** *(Melaleuca leucadendron)*

*Blends well with:*
juniper
hyssop
sandalwood

This is an essential oil from a small branch of the Myrtaceae family called *Melaleuca* and is steam distilled from the leaves and buds of the cajuput, which grows wild in the Far East. (It can also be spelt cajeput.)

Circulatory: haemorrhoids, varicose veins
Digestive: gastro-enteritis, colic, colitis
Excretory: cystitis, urethritis
Head: colds, earache, laryngitis, sinusitis, toothache
Menstrual: painful periods
Muscular: aches and pains, arthritis, rheumatism
Nervous: facial neuralgia
Respiratory: asthma, chronic bronchitis, coughs, 'flu, pharygnitis
Skin: insect repellent, inflammatory skin conditions, psoriasis
Special: gout

**Caraway** *(Carum carvi)*

*Blends well with:*
aniseed
cinnamon
peppermint

The essential oil is distilled from the crushed seeds of the caraway. It is one of the few oils obtained mainly from European countries and the plant is related to fennel and dill – all are from the Umbelliferae family.

Digestive: flatulence, gastric spasm, indigestion, loss of appetite
Head: hay fever, vertigo (dizziness), scalp problems (stimulant)
Nervous: anger
Respiratory: bronchitis

**Clary-Sage** *(Salvia sclarea)*

*Blends well with:*
ccdarwood
citrus oils
frankincense
geranium
jasmine
juniper
lavender
sandalwood

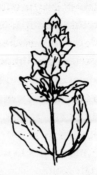

Clary-sage is another Lamiate and should not be confused with sage, a different size of plant, growing 2–3 times as high as sage, and having different properties. Russia has the largest output of clary-sage oil, though small amounts are produced in Morocco and the South of France. It has high fixative powers and the flowering tops and foliage of this beautiful 4–5 ft plant are used to extract the oil. The word 'clary' originates from the Latin for 'clear', because an eye lotion used to be made from the seeds of this plant. Dry soil, high elevation, shade from olive trees, sun and *spring* rain give a much superior oil than that from rich moist soil at low levels. Quality also varies according to use of manure, the time of day of picking, the dryness of the plant, and whether the seeds are completely formed. Known in Germany as Muscatel sage; together with elder flowers it was used in the making of German 'Muscatel' wines. Used by the Italians in various brands of vermouth. Now an invaluable ingredient of eau-de-colognes and lavender water.

Circulatory: circulatory problems, haemorrhoids, varicose
    veins

Head: alopecia
Menstrual: irregularity, painful and difficult periods, lack of
   periods, menopause, PMS
Nervous: nervous anxiety and tension, nervous debility
Skin: fungal conditions, inflamed, mature (ageing), sweating

## Coriander *(Coriandrum sativum)*

*Blends well with:*
bergamot
ginger
nutmeg

Coriander is a steam distilled oil and the essential oil is
obtained from the seeds. It is a member of the Apiaceae family and it is an excellent stimulant of the digestive and nervous
systems.

Digestive: indigestion, flatulence, sluggish digestion, gastro-
   enteritis
Excretory: cystitis
Muscular: aches and pains, arthritis, rheumatism
Nervous: anorexia, apathy, debility, mental fatigue, nervous
   exhaustion, sadness (tonic)

## Eucalyptus – Blue Gum *(Eucalyptus globulus)*

*Blends well with:*
benzoin
lavender
pine

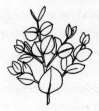

Belonging to the Myrtaceae family this oil is obtained from the fresh leaves, which are rich in essential oil. Although eucalyptus is one of the tallest trees in the world, trees are kept beheaded to make branches more accessible. Grown in China, Tasmania, Africa, Portugal and France, there are about 200 species of eucalyptus. Has been used to rub countless chests over the years, to improve breathing in colds and sinusitis, and has a definite cooling effect on body temperature – a febrifuge.

Excretory: cystitis

Head: colds, congestive headache, laryngitis, migraine, sinusitis, throat infections

Muscular: aches and pains, rheumatoid arthritis, sprains

Nervous: neuralgia

Respiratory: asthma, bronchitis, catarrh, coughs, 'flu, infections

Skin: good antiseptic, herpes, ulcers, wounds, insect repellent

Special: candida, thrush

*Note:* Do not use on babies or very young children as the oil is often adulterated, making it too powerful for them. A much better eucalyptus to use is gully gum eucalyptus (*Eucalyptus Smithii* – see below), which is a much gentler oil and can be applied neat in the first application for a chesty cough or bronchitis, to give it a 'kick-start'.

## Eucalyptus – Gully Gum *(Eucalyptus Smithii)*

This gentle eucalyptus has great synergistic powers and is very beneficial to use in a blend with others, as well as on its own; it is especially useful for use by the whole family over the winter period, to help prevent the usual run of coughs and colds.

Digestive: stimulant to the digestive process
Head: colds, congestive headaches
Muscular: aches and pains (including due to sprains), rheuma-
 toid arthritis
Nervous: calming (evening use)
Respiratory: asthma, bronchitis, coughs, 'flu

**Lemon** *(Citrus limon)*

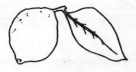

*Blends well with:*
lavender
neroli

Another citrus oil from the Rutaceae family, lemon is obtained
from the rind of the fruit, like bergamot. The Arabians introduced the lemon to Europe, and the tree was first grown in
California in 1887. The trees attain a height of 12 to 15 feet
(3.5 to 4.5m) and bear great quantities of fruit. The principal
seat of the lemon oil industry is Sicily, though the most modern techniques of production are carried out in California,
Florida and the island of Cyprus. In Italy the fruit used to be
halved by children and women scraped out the flesh; the peel
was then steeped for a few minutes in cold water and the next
day men sponge-pressed the peel. The oil squeezed from the
sponges was left to settle, then decanted and filtered. Mechan-
ical methods are mostly used nowadays, but the hand
processed oil, still done in some parts, is the better quality.

Circulatory: anaemia, chilblains, poor circulation, varicose
 veins, high blood pressure
Digestive: diabetes, diarrhoea, flatulence, gallstones, gastro-
 enteritis, loss of appetite, nausea, painful digestion, vomiting, stomach ulcers

Excretory: fluid retention (diuretic), obesity, oedema, stones

Head: colds, greasy scalp, herpes (cold sore), nose bleeds, headache, sinusitis, sore throat

Muscular: arthritis, rheumatism

Nervous: insomnia, nightmares

Respiratory: asthma, bronchitis, nervous excitability, catarrh, 'flu

Skin: boils, broken capillaries, congestion in tissues, greasy skin, insect bites, wrinkles (ageing), warts, veruccas

Special: gout, low immune system

### Lemongrass *(Cymbopogon citratus)*

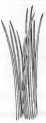

*Blends well with:*
geranium
jasmine
lavender

Belonging to the Poaceae family, lemongrass oil is obtained by distillation from two species of grasses which grow wild and are also cultivated in Madras, Malay, the West Indies. Distillation takes place from July to January and about 100 kilos of grass are needed to yield 21 kgs of oil. It is one of the largest production essential oils – over 2000 tons a year being distilled. The oil is the colour of dry sherry and has a lemonish smell which is very powerful.

Digestive: colitis, sluggish digestion, gastro-enteritis

Head: lice, vertigo (dizziness)

Muscular: poor tone, slack tissue

Nervous: palpitations

Skin: acne and open pores, insect repellent, tonic

*Note:* Lemongrass should be used with care as it is a skin irritant, therefore do not use neat. Do not use on babies or children.

**Niaouli** *(Melaleuca viridiflora)*

*Blends well with:*
geranium
lavender
patchouli
tea tree

Occasionally called gomenol, this oil is distilled from the leaves. It belongs to the *Melaleuca* branch of the Myrtaceae family and in the country of origin it is used as lavender is in this country, for almost everything!

Circulatory: haemorrhoids, high blood pressure, varicose veins
Digestive: indigestion, gastro-enteritis, colitis, diarrhoea, gall stones
Head: colds, sore throat, sinusitis
Menstrual: irregular periods, lack of periods
Muscular: rheumatoid arthritis
Respiratory: bronchitis, catarrh, chest infections, coughs
Skin: fungal infections, boils, insect bites, psoriasis, ulcers, infected wounds
Special: low immune system

**Orange** *(Citrus aurantium var. amara; C. aurantium var. sinensis)*

*Blends well with:*
cedarwood
geranium
ginger
petitgrain

Orange oil is the name given to the essential oil expressed from the peel of the fruit (the other two oils, petitgrain and neroli, are distilled from the leaves and flowers respectively), *amara* yielding bitter orange oil and *sinensis*, sweet orange oil. Thought to have originated in southern China, the orange tree found its way to southern Europe and later to America and Brazil (the bitter orange tree being first). Sweet orange oil has milder effects than bitter orange and is very suitable for children. Beware a clear orange oil as this means the oranges have been distilled and their oil is not so suitable for aromatherapy – the quality of the expressed oil is much superior. Good digestive oils, both bitter and sweet orange oils are beneficial to the skin, bitter orange being more helpful to oily skin and prevention of ageing.

Circulation: poor circulation (stimulating)
Digestive: constipation, indigestion, gastric spasms
Head: vertigo (dizziness)
Nervous: anxiety, insomnia, palpitations
Skin: mouth ulcers, oily

**Petitgrain** *(Citrus aurantium* var. *amara)*

*Blends well with:*
lavender
lemon
geranium

The best petitgrain (usually from South America, France and North Africa) is distilled from the leaves of the bitter orange tree (the flowers of which produce neroli), though an oil of lesser quality can be obtained from a mixture of leaves and twigs. Like all citrus fruits, petitgrain belongs to the Rutaceae family. The better the quality, the nearer the aroma is to neroli although it never quite matches neroli, which is a superb essential oil. Petitgrain is an excellent oil to balance the skin.

Nervous: relaxing when better quality oil is used, promotes sleep, relieves apathy and irritability
Respiratory: infections
Skin: acne, boils, oily

**Sage** *(Salvia officinalis)*

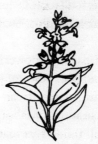

*Blends well with:*
bergamot
lemon
lavender
rosemary

This member of the Lamiaceae family has its oils extracted from leaves which are sometimes dried in the hot sun before distilling. It is comparatively expensive because of the hard labour involved in preparation. The herb is indigenous to the countries bordering the northern coasts of the Mediterranean. It is a yellow oil with a strong, herby smell. Sometimes used to adulterate rosemary and spike lavender oils. Sage tea, regularly taken for four weeks before childbirth, can help to relieve labour pains and also helps to reduce fluid retention and obesity.

Circulation: low blood pressure, poor circulation, sluggish lymph

Digestive: loss of appetite, sluggish digestion, indigestion, liver stimulant

Excretory: diuretic (fluid retention), urinary disorders

Head: alopecia, sinusitis, sore throat, toothache

Menstrual: irregular periods, lack of, or scanty periods, menopause, ovary problems, painful and difficult periods, vaginal discharge

Muscular: all rheumatic conditions, aches and pains in joints

Nervous: general debility (good nerve tonic)

Respiratory: asthma, bronchitis, 'flu

Skin: cellulite, genital herpes, insect bites, sluggish or congested (tonic), shingles, sweating

Special: candida, facilitates delivery in childbirth, thrush

*Note:* Sage is a powerful oil and should be used with discretion and advice. Best not used during pregnancy except for the last month, when it can help tone and strengthen the uterus in preparation for labour. At this time, use under the direction of a well trained aromatherapist or an aromatologist.

**Tea Tree** *(Melaleuca alternifolia)*

*Blends well with:*
chamomile
lemon
myrrh

This oil is not produced anywhere except Australia, and is steam distilled locally from the leaves and small branches. Tea tree belongs to the *Melaleuca* branch of the Myrtaceae family. The name 'tea' is not to be confused with the tea we drink and is supposed to originate from the day Captain Cook landed in Australia. His men had had no tea to drink for days and having made a cup of 'tea' with the leaves of a tree which was growing in abundance, they named the tree 'tea tree' even though there was no resemblance in taste to the tea imported at that time from India and China. Tea tree is a strong antiseptic.

Circulatory: haemorrhoids, varicose veins
Digestive: viral enteritis, worms
Head: mouth infections, sinusitis, sore throat
Menstrual: PMS
Nervous: anxiety, debility, depression, PMS
Respiratory: bronchitis
Skin: abcesses, acne, candida, infected wounds, insect bites
Special: candida, low immune system

**Thyme** *(Thymus vulgaris)*

Thyme oil is obtained from the whole leafy parts of the plants by steam distillation. *Thymus vulgaris* (a Lamiate) produces identical looking plants having different principal components, divisible roughly into phenolic and sweet thymes.

Sweet thymes contain mostly alcohols, phenolic ones containing predominantly phenols which are harsh. The two types of oil are completely different, a sweet thyme being able to be used on children and a phenolic thyme needing care in use because of its high phenol content. When thyme plants are grown from the *seeds* of either phenolic or sweet thymes, the plants which grow are a mixture of all six types of *T. vulgaris*. The essential oil from a field of these plants is called 'population thyme' and contains both phenols and alcohols. To obtain a specific phenolic or sweet thyme, it is necessary to identify plants and grow what you want from cuttings. This is called *cloning*.

When buying thyme essential oil, always ask whether it contains phenols or alcohols. If the vendor does not know – and the oil is cheap – it will be a phenolic thyme, as this is more readily available from retail shops. It is better to buy essential oils from someone who knows the difference, as the quality will also be better.

*Phenolic Thyme (Carvacrol and thymol clones)*

*Blends well with:*
geranium
lavandin
rosemary
sandalwood

Phenolic thyme is used extensively in cooking as well as in medicine; it is a very strong antiseptic and is effective in the control of many parasites. It is said to stimulate the production of white corpuscles in the blood in infectious diseases and is also an excellent nerve tonic.

Circulatory: anaemia, low blood pressure
Digestive: flatulence, sluggish digestion
Excretory: cystitis
Head: colds, coughs, alopecia (hair loss), mental stimulant,
    sinusitis, sore throat
Muscular: rheumatism
Nervous: anxiety, depression, nervous debility, sciatica
Respiratory: asthma, bronchitis, 'flu
Skin: abscesses, acne, boils, infected wounds
Special: intestinal parasites, lice, nits

*Note:* Phenolic thymes should be used with care under the
direction of an aromatherapist as they irritate the skin in too
strong a concentration. Do not use on children and babies.
Sweet thymes (see below) are the *only* choice when thyme oil is
needed on children. They are by far the gentlest on the skin, yet
share many important properties with the phenolic thymes.

*Sweet Thyme (linalool, geraniol, thujanol clones)*

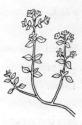

*Blends well with:*
bergamot
lemon
melissa
rosemary

Sweet thyme has many therapeutic properties, being helpful
for headaches, especially nervous headaches. It is a gentle and
effective oil and can be used with safety on young children.

Digestive: colitis, diabetes, gastro-enteritis (antiviral), slug-
    gish liver
Excretory: cystitis, diuretic, urinary tract infections

Head: colds, earache (inflammation), sinusitis, sore throat, tonsillitis
Muscular: arthritis, aches and pains, tendonitis, rheumatism
Nervous: anxiety, fatigue, insomnia
Respiratory: asthma, bronchitis, 'flu
Skin: infected acne, dermatitis, eczema (weeping and dry), verrucae
Special: candida, facilitates delivery in childbirth, low immune system

## MIDDLE NOTES

These affect most body systems and general metabolism.

**Aniseed** *(Pimpinella anisum)*

*Blends well with:*
coriander
lemon
peppermint

Aniseed is from the Apiaceae family and is well known as an ingredient in some aperitifs. This oil is obtained by distillation of the seeds of the plant and is used in medical preparations to help digestion. It is produced in many countries but it was first used in the Middle East.

Digestive: colic, flatulence, loss of appetite, nervous indigestion, nervous vomiting
Excretory: diuretic
Head: migraine, vertigo (dizziness)
Menstrual: lack of periods, menopause, painful periods, PMS
Muscular: aches and pains, arthritis, rheumatism

Nervous: palpitations, sciatica
Respiratory: asthma, bronchitis, catarrhal congestion, coughs, difficulty in breathing
Special: facilitates delivery in childbirth, lack of milk

*Note:* Care and advice should be taken with this oil because of its high phenolic ether content. Do not use during pregnancy until labour commences.

**Black Pepper** *(Piper nigrum)*

*Blends well with:*
frankincense
juniper
lemon
sandalwood

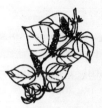

The pepper plant, which belongs to the family Piperaceae, is a climber which clings to trees for shade and support. The spike of unripe berries is picked and they change from red to black as they dry in the sun. Only a very small proportion of the yield of black pepper is made into essential oil, and the commercial centre for this oil is Singapore. In Nossi Be and the Comoro Islands oil is distilled on the spot and often a good quality oil is produced. A green-yellow oil of great pungency.

Circulatory: stimulating (rubefacient)
Digestive: colic, food poisoning, indigestion, sluggish digestion, sluggish liver
Excretory: urinary system, antiseptic
Head: colds, headache caused by cold in head, high temperature, laryngitis, toothache

Muscular: aches and pains, lack of tone
Respiratory: catarrh, chronic bronchitis, coughs


**Chamomile** *(Chamaemelum nobile* – Roman; *Chamomilla recutita* – German; *Ormenis mixta* – Moroccan)*

*Blends well with:*
geranium
lavender
patchouli
rose otto

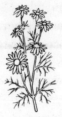

There are three plants with the common name 'chamomile' and all belong to the Asteraceae family. Roman chamomile is distilled from the dried flowers of *Chamaemelum nobile*. Used a lot because of its azulene content, which is not present in the flower but forms as the essential oil is distilled out of the plant. Chamomile changes with exposure to light and air from blue to browny-yellow. Roman chamomile produced in Belgium is light blue-green-yellowy brown. In England the centre for this oil is Long Melford. German chamomile (from Germany, Hungary, Russia and Slovakia) is deep blue and contains more azulene. It is distilled from *Chamomilla recutita*. Moroccan chamomile is obtained from *Ormenis mixta* which is grown wild; it is not a true chamomile. Chamomile is helpful for most disorders and has a very low toxicity, therefore is very useful for treating children. Chamomile flower heads are used in shampoos to lighten blonde hair.

The properties of each chamomile are slightly different. As a guide the table below shows the variety of chamomile (in brackets) most likely to help the problem.

Digestive: colic (R), colitis (M), diarrhoea (in children – R), flatulence (R), gastric spasm (G), gastritis (G), indigestion – especially in children (G&R), nausea (morning sickness – G), sluggish liver (M), loss of appetite (R), gastric ulcers (G), stomach ulcers (G)

Excretory: cystitis (M)

Head: headache (R), migraine (R),

Menstrual: irregularity (R), lack of periods (G&R), menopause (R), painful (G&R), PMS (G)

Muscular: all aches and pains – especially after sport, arthritis and rheumatism (G, M&R)

Nervous: depression (M&R), insomnia (R), irritability (R), tantrums – in children (R)

Skin: acne (R&M), boils (G&M), burns (G&R), cysts (M), dermatitis (M&R), eczema (G, M&R), inflammation (G, M&R), irritability (M&R), wounds (R), ulcers (G)

Special: gout (R)

**Cypress** *(Cupressus sempervirens)*

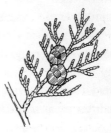

*Blends well with:*
juniper
lavender
pine
sandalwood

A member of the Cupressaceae family, cypress (distilled from the leavy twigs in Germany and France) produces an oil which can be compared with witch hazel and horse-chestnut in its effects. It is said to be superior to witch hazel (*Hamamelis*) which, according to Steffen Arctander, has no therapeutic use! The oil is slightly yellow. Cypress oil is also

produced in Kenya and Spain from *Cupressus lusitanica* and this
too is used medicinally.

Circulatory: broken veins, haemorrhoids, sluggish circulation,
    varicose veins
Excretory: bedwetting, diuretic, fluid retention
Head: nose bleed
Menstrual: excessive loss, ovary problems
Muscular: cramp, rheumatic swelling
Nervous: excitability, irritability, debility
Respiratory: asthma, bronchitis, 'flu, spasmodic cough
Skin: broken capillaries, bruises, sweating

### Fennel (Sweet) *(Foeniculum vulgare* var. *dulce)*

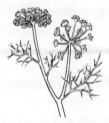

*Blends well with:*
geranium
lavender
rose otto
sandalwood

There is a bitter and a sweet fennel in the Apiaceae family, but
only sweet fennel is used in aromatherapy (and aperitifs).
Sweet fennel is widely grown throughout the world – the
Mediterranean, India, Asia, America and Europe. It has a
pleasant sweet aroma reminiscent of aniseed, and is tradition-
ally used in cooking, especially with fish. Because of its effect
on the hormones, and its diuretic qualities, it is an invaluable
oil for reducing obesity. It is also well known for its aid to
digestive problems (used in gripewater for babies).

Digestive: constipation, flatulence, food poisoning (preventative), gastro-enteritis, indigestion, loss of appetite, stomach pains

Excretory: cystitis, diuretic, fluid retention (obesity), kidney stones, urinary tract infections

Menstrual: lack of periods, irregular periods, painful periods, menopausal irregularities, ovary problems, PMS

Nervous: palpitations

Respiratory: hiccups, rapid breathing

Skin: cellulite, mature oedema

Special: facilitates delivery in childbirth, gout, lack of milk

*Note:* Fennel is a powerful oil because of its phenolic ether content. It should be used with care or advice and not during pregnancy until labour commences.

**Geranium** *(Pelargonium graveolens)*

*Blends well with nearly all oils, especially:*
basil
citrus oils
rose otto

Geranium from the Geranaceae family, is an easy oil to adulterate. Reunion (formerly Ile de Bourbon) used to produce the most oil, and it is steam distilled from the leaves of the *Pelargonium* plant. It is also grown extensively in France, Africa, Spain, Italy, China and Corsica in frost-free areas.

Circulatory: decongestant (breasts and lymph), haemorrhoids, varicose veins

Digestive: colic, colitis, diabetes, diarrhoea, gastro-enteritis, jaundice, sluggish liver, stomach ulcers

Excretory: fluid retention, mild diuretic, urinary tract disorders

Head: throat and mouth infections, tonsillitis

Menstrual: painful periods, leucorrhoea, PMS

Muscular: arthritis, cramp, rheumatism

Nervous: agitation, anxiety, debility, depression, neuralgia, nervous fatigue

Skin: acne, athlete's foot, burns, cellulite, chapped and cracked, cleansing, cuts, dermatitis, dry eczema, impetigo, infections, inflamed, insect repellent, oedema, oily, shingles, stretch marks, tonic, ulcers, wounds

Special: candida

## Hyssop *(Hyssopus officinalis)*

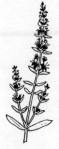

*Blends well with:*
citrus oils
clary-sage
lavender
rosemary
sage

Another oil from the large Lamiaceae family, hyssop is well known for its medicinal uses, and is excellent as a tonic. The oil is obtained from cultivated plants in Provence and Germany, and is often used in eau-de-cologne. The Hebrews called this plant Ezob and our name for hyssop stems from this: 'Purge me with hyssop and I shall be clean', Psalm 51:9 (actually, the hyssop in the Bible is a different plant). It is especially good for asthma and related problems, in fact any respiratory problem. It is a small plant with thin leaves and small, usually blue flowers, both of which are used in distillation to obtain essential oil.

Circulatory: low blood pressure
Digestive: sluggish digestion, loss of appetite, mild laxative
Excretory: cystitis, diuretic, kidney stones
Head: colds, hay fever, sinusitis
Mesntrual: leucorrhoea, irregular periods, scanty periods
Muscular: rheumatism, sprains
Nervous: general debility
Respiratory: asthma, bronchitis, catarrh, coughs and 'flu
Skin: bruises, dermatitis, eczema, scars, wounds

*Note:* Hyssop is a powerful oil and should be used with care. It should not be used during pregnancy nor by people prone to epilepsy.

## Juniper *(Juniperus communis)*

*Blends well with:*
benzoin
cypress
lavender
sandalwood

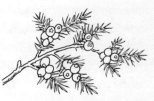

The juniper tree is a member of the Cupressaceae family and juniper oil is distilled from the dried fruits of the juniper bush, which grows in Europe and Canada. The oil is colourless or pale yellow and grows darker and thicker with age and exposure to air. Used to flavour gin. Known since ancient times for its antiseptic and diuretic qualities. It is very useful in worried or anxious states of mind.

Digestive: diabetes, loss of appetite
Excretory: cystitis, diuretic, fluid retention, urinary stones
Head: greasy scalp
Muscular: rheumatic pain
Nervous: debility, fatigue (tonic)
Skin: acne, cellulite, dermatitis, eczema, oedema, oily
Special: gout

**Lavandin** *(Lavandula x intermedia)*

*Blends well with many oils (as does lavender), especially:*
eucalyptus
geranium
petitgrain

A member of the Lamiaceae family, lavandin is a hybrid of
true lavender and spike lavender (an enormous plant yielding
much oil, though often camphoraceous). There are many
different lavandins with varying properties, depending on the
individual original lavender and spike lavender plants chosen
to be crossed. Each crossing of these plants resulted in a
stronger and bigger plant than lavender, but the oil still contained more camphor and did not quite reach the sweet flow-
ery aroma of true lavender. However, lavandin has greatly
replaced lavender in the perfume industry because of the lower cost and is often passed off as fine lavender. Very useful for
soaps and cosmetics, a good quality lavandin has several therapeutic characteristics similar to lavender and its camphor
content makes it superior for rheumatism.

Digestive: gastro-enteritis
Head: chronic migraine, sore throat
Muscular: muscular pain, rheumatism

Nervous: debility, depression, listlessness
Respiratory: bronchitis, coughs
Skin: acne, athlete's foot, greasy, wounds
Special: candida

**Lavender** *(Lavandula angustifolia; L. officinalis or L. vera)*

*Blends well with most oils, especially:*
citrus oils
clary-sage
patchouli
pine
rosemary

This oil is the most used and perhaps the most versatile of all the essential oils. A Lamiate, it is distilled from *Lavandula angustifolia* Miller; plants are rarely grown from seed, but from cuttings of the strongest plants from the *L. officinalis, L. angustifolia* or *L. vera*, all three names are synonymous botanically. The best lavender comes from France, the mountainous areas of Provence, though cloned lavender (having far fewer constituents) is grown in Australia, Bulgaria and former Yugoslavia. Oil glands are embedded among the tiny hairs with which the flowers, leaves and stems are covered, and the aroma has a comparatively short life. Lavender used to be subject to extensive adulteration, but now lavandin and spike lavender are used instead of lavender in soaps, household goods and cheaper perfumes, leaving lavender for therapeutic use and the better quality perfumes. Unfortunately it is still adulterated with lavandin (as demand is always greater than supply) and a true lavender should be bought from someone who knows the source – and sometimes even the farmer! It is a very useful oil (like chamomile) especially when symptoms are due to a nervous problem:

Circulatory: chilblains, lowers high blood pressure
Digestive: colic, flatulence
Excretory: cystitis
Head: dry scalp, earache, headache, migraine, nose and throat infections, sinusitis
Menstrual: irregularity, leucorrhoea, scanty periods, PMS
Muscular: aches and pains, arthritis, cramp, rheumatism, sprains
Nervous: anxiety, depression, excitability, general debility, insomnia, irritability, palpitations, sleep problems
Respiratory: all catarrhal complaints, 'flu, spasmodic cough
Skin: acne (rosacea, juvenile), athlete's foot, bites, boils, bruises, burns, dermatitis, dry, dry eczema, herpes, inflammation, insect bites, itchiness, mature, oily, psoriasis, regenerative, sunburn, varicose ulcers
Special: candida

### Marjoram (Sweet) *(Origanum majorana)*

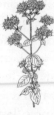

*Blends well with:*
bergamot
lavender
rosemary

Distilled from the flowering heads of sweet marjoram, this Lamiate grows in Spain, southern France and Tunisia. It was grown and used in ancient times by the Egyptians. The oil is colourless with a persistent odour. A very 'comforting' oil if low in spirits. Always buy this oil by its Latin name as Spanish marjoram (*Thymus mastichina*), which is sold as marjoram, is not a marjoram at all, but a variety of thyme, and has different properties and effects.

Circulatory: fainting, lowers high blood pressure
Digestive: colic, diarrhoea, flatulence, indigestion, relieves
  spasm in intestines
Head: colds in the head, headache, migraine, sinusitis,
  toothache, vertigo (dizziness)
Muscular: all muscular pain, arthritis, cramp, rheumatism,
  spasm, sprains
Nervous: agitation, anguish, anxiety, calmative, general debility, insomnia, irritability, palpitations
Respiratory: asthma, bronchitis, catarrh, coughs, respiratory
  infections

### Melissa (True) *(Melissa officinalis)*

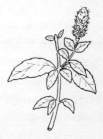

*Blends well with:*
geranium
lavender
neroli
ylang-ylang

The local name in southern Europe is 'heart's delight', and it is often called the 'elixir of life'. It has been used medicinally since the seventeenth century, and is a very cheering oil, making a good general tonic. This Lamiate is also known as lemon balm oil, and is obtained by distilling the leaves and tops, which contain very little essential oil – the reason why the true oil is so expensive.

Circulation: lowers high blood pressure
Digestive: indigestion, nausea, morning sickness, sluggish
    liver, stomach cramp
Head: headache, migraine, vertigo (dizziness)
Menstrual: irregular, lack of periods, painful, PMS, scanty
Nervous: agitation, insomnia, nervous tension, palpitations
Skin: cold stores, mature, regenerating, shingles, bee stings

### Peppermint *(Menthax* x *piperita)*

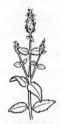

*Blends well with:*
aniseed
benzoin
lemon
rosemary

Peppermint is yet another oil from the Lamiaceae family, distilled from the leaves and flowering tops. It is cultivated in
Europe, USA and Japan, but English oil is reputed to be the
best. It is widely used in confectionery and toiletry as well as
being an excellent therapeutic oil. Use in a tea instead of
aspirin – much healthier for your stomach.

Circulatory: low blood pressure
Digestive: colic, colitis, flatulence, gastric spasm, gastro-
    enteritis, heartburn, indigestion, irritable bowel syndrome,
    jaundice, sluggish liver, stomach pains, travel sickness,
    nervous (vomiting)
Excretory: cystitis
Head: bad breath, colds, headache, laryngitis, migraine
    (digestive origin), sinusitis
Menstrual: hot flushes, irregular periods (ovarian stimulant)
Nervous: apathy (neurotonic)

Respiratory: bronchial asthma, bronchitis
Skin: broken capillaries, herpes (cold sore), irritation, inflammation, nettle rash, rashes, sunburn (less than 1%), sweating (hot flushes), urticaria
Special: facilitates delivery in childbirth, too much milk

**Pine Needle** *(Pinus sylvestris)*

*Blends well with:*
cedarwood
lavender
petitgrain
rosemary

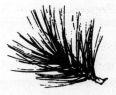

Pine comes from the Pinaceae family (a branch of the Conifer class). Distilled from the needles and cones, good oils are obtained from north east Russia and the Austrian Tyrol. Used extensively in soaps, bath preparations and, because of its antiseptic qualities, in detergents, etc.

Circulatory: low blood pressure, sluggish lymph
Digestive: diabetes, gall stones, stomach pains
Excretory: cystitis, urinary infections
Head: colds, sinusitis
Menstrual: pain due to uterine or ovarian congestion
Muscular: arthritis, rheumatism
Nervous: general debility, fatigue
Respiratory: all infections of respiratory tract, asthma, bronchitis, coughs, 'flu
Skin: inflammation, sweating of the feet
Special: gout

**Rosemary** *(Rosmarinus officinalis)*

*Blends well with:*
basil
cedarwood
citrus oils
frankincense
lavender
peppermint

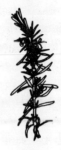

Rosemary, a well-known *Lamiate*, is distilled from the flowering tops and leaves of *Rosmarinus officinalis*, and is grown in countries bordering the Mediterranean, chiefly southern France, Spain and the Dalmation Islands (garden legend has it that 'where rosemary thrives the mistress is master'). The quality of oil from Spain varies from very high to very low and oil of the most consistently high qualities comes from Tunisia. It is possible to adulterate rosemary oil with turpentine, sage and spike oils. Rosemary has been used in eau-de-cologne. It has been in therapeutic use for hundreds of years.

Circulatory: regulates blood pressure (depending on dose), lymphatic congestion, poor circulation
Digestive: colitis, constipation, diarrhoea (balancing), flatulence, gall stones, gastro-enteritis, indigestion, jaundice, liver problems, sluggish digestion, stomach pains
Excretory: bedwetting, cystitis, diuretic, fluid retention
Head: alopecia, colds, dandruff, earache, headache, migraine, memory loss, scalp disorders, sinusitis
Menstrual: lack of periods, scanty periods
Muscular: aches and pains, cramp, rheumatism, sprains, stiffness

Nervous: agitation, fainting, general debility, loss of nerve
   function, paralysis, mental fatigue, mental strain, nerve
   tonic, neuralgia, palpitations
Respiratory: asthma, chronic bronchitis, coughs, 'flu
Skin: bruises, burns, cellulite, congestion, wounds
Special: candida, gout

*Note:* Rosemary oils containing a high proportion of camphor
or other ketones should not be used during pregnancy.

**Savory** *(Satureia montana)*

*Blends well with:*
black pepper
coriander
clove bud

From the Lamiaceae family again, savory is distilled from the
leaves and flowering tops of the plant. It is very aromatic and
was renowned in the past for its culinary properties, as indeed
it is today.

Circulatory: low blood pressure
Digestive: colic, colitis, diarrhoea, sluggish or painful
   digestion
Excretory: cystitis
Head: fungal infections of the mouth, sore throat
Muscular: arthritis, rheumatism
Nervous: debility, depression (tonic), mental fatigue
Respiratory: asthma, bronchitis, catarrh, coughs
Skin: abcesses, impetigo, infections, insect bites, sores
Special: candida, low immune system

*Note:* Use with care, as savory is a skin irritant which contains a phenol called carvacrol.


## BASE NOTES

All base notes are sedative.

**Benzoin** a resinoid (*Styrax tonkinensis*)

*Blends well with:*
cedarwood
petitgrain
rose otto
sandalwood

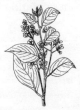

Benzoin, a member of the Styracaceae family, is collected as a resin exuded from the trunk after the bark is cut, and is in solid brown to white brittle pieces. More processing is required to bring the benzoin to liquid form; it is not distilled so it is not an essential oil. Benzoin comes from trees native to Thailand and Sumatra, and is an ingredient of incense. Commonly known as 'friar's balsam'.

Circulatory: stimulating
Joints: rheumatoid arthritis
Nervous: emotional exhaustion, tension
Respiratory: asthma, bronchitis, catarrh, coughs, 'flu (lung antiseptic)
Skin: burns, chapped, cracked, cuts, dry, dermatitis, eczema, irritable, mature, psoriasis, wounds
Special: gout

*Note:* As it is not distilled oil, do not ingest. Care should also be taken to obtain a good quality oil, so as not to initiate a skin rash – possible with a poor quality oil.

## **Cedarwood** *(Cedrus atlantica)*

*Blends well with:*
bergamot
cypress
jasmine
juniper
neroli
rosemary

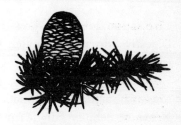

One of the earliest essential oils, used in the preservation of mummies, cedarwood is obtained by steam distillation from the wood of this member of the Pinaceae family. It has been used for many years by natives for medicinal purposes.

Circulation: sluggish lymph
Excretory: cystitis, difficulty or pain, fluid retention
Head: alopecia, dandruff, seborrhoea of scalp and hair
Respiratory: bronchitis, catarrh, coughs
Skin: acne, cellulite, eczema, insect repellent, irritation, oily, seborrhoea of scalp

## **Clove** *(Syzygium aromaticum)*

*Blends well with:*
juniper
sage
sweet thyme

The best clove essential oil is distilled from the flower buds. The spice was highly valued in the nineteenth century – so much so that clove merchants became the first American millionaires. Zambia is the best known country for cloves (which belong to the Myrtaceae family), though they are grown in several other countries including Madagascar and the West Indies.

Circulation: low blood pressure
Digestive: diarrhoea, flatulence, gastro-enteritis, gastric spasm
Excretory: cystitis
Head: sinusitis, toothache
Muscular: arthritis, rheumatism (pain)
Nervous: debility, fatigue (mental and general), memory loss, neuralgia
Respiratory: asthma, bronchitis
Skin: abcesses, infected acne, insect repellent, ulcers, wounds
Special: difficult or long labour in childbirth, low immune system

*Note:* Use with care or advice, as it is a powerful oil.

**Frankincense** *(Boswellia carteri)*

*Blends well with:*
basil
black pepper
camphor
citrus oils
geranium
lavender
pine
sandalwood

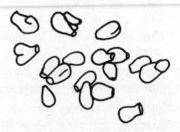

Frankincense (olibanum) is a whitish gum which has to be dissolved and distilled to produce essential oil. The trees, which are members of the Burseraceae family, grow in East Africa and the aromatic resin permeates the bark. (Used in Egyptian times in rejuvenating face masks.) This, with myrrh, was first used as incense and is produced mainly in Iran and Lebanon. Was once highly valuable, hence the offering to baby Jesus.

Muscular: rheumatic pain, sprains
Nervous: anxiety, depression (energizing), tension
Respiratory: asthma, bronchitis, catarrh and other mucous
  conditions
Skin: inflamed, mature (ageing), poor tonicity, regenerative,
  scars, ulcers, wounds
Special: low immune system

## Ginger *(Zingiber officinale)*

*Blends well with:*
coriander
lemon
nutmeg

Ginger, whose family name is Zingerberaceae, is distilled from the roots of the plant and is used in herbal medicine and cooking mainly for its digestive properties.

Circulation: stimulating
Digestive: constipation, diarrhoea (balancing), flatulence, loss
  of appetite, indigestion, nausea, sluggish digestion
Head: sore throat, toothache
Muscular: aches and pains, rheumatism
Nervous: fatigue, general nerve tonic
Respiratory: chronic bronchitis

**Jasmine** – an absolute *(Jasminum grandiflorum)*

*Blends well with all oils, especially*
citrus oils

Jasmine is not an essential oil; it is obtained by means of sol-vents or enfleurage from the flowers of this exotic plant, whose family name is Oleaceae. The best absolute is extracted by means of the solvent ether and, although a good quality oil is very expensive, much *less* is needed to give the desired effect; therefore it is economical in use and can be used where the aroma is the most important consideration. It is most effective on the nervous system, and is invaluable for symp-toms with a psychological and psychosomatic origin. Great care is needed when buying jasmine oil as 90 per cent of jas-mines on the market are adulterated in some way, many with synthetic substances. These last are not suitable for aromather-apy, not least because they could irritate or cause a skin rash.

Menstrual: pain of any kind
Nervous: apathy, depression, listlessness, nervous debility, sedative and uplifting
Skin: (quality oil only), irritable, sensitive
Special: childbirth (aroma relaxing), lack of milk

*Note:* This is not an essential oil, therefore do not ingest.

**Myrrh** *(Commiphora myrrha)*

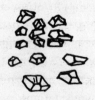

*Blends well with:*
camphor
lavender

Myrrh is a gum resin which naturally exudes from the trunk of this member of the Burseraceae family, which is then distilled for the essential oil. Used in rejuvenating face masks during Egyptian times, and also for embalming. Mentioned in ancient history (about 1700 BC). When Joseph was sold by his brothers to the Ishmaelite caravan, their camels were carrying gum, balm and myrrh to Egypt. Myrrh is a hormonal oil and is said to be a sexual tonic.

Digestive: aids digestion, flatulence
Excretory: antiseptic to urinary tract
Head: laryngitis, mouth ulcers, pyorrhoea
Menstrual: leucorrhoea
Respiratory: all types of discharges, bronchitis, 'flu, soothes
    respiratory tract
Skin: anti-inflammatory, boils, mature, regenerating, skin diseases, sores, ulcers, wounds

**Neroli** *(Citrus aurantium var. amara)*

*Blends well with most oils, especially:*
benzoin
clary-sage
geranium
lavender

This exotic oil distilled from the flowers of the bitter orange tree may be called 'neroli' because the wife of a famous prince in Nerola, Italy, used it to perfume her bath water and her gloves. (The oil distilled from sweet orange flowers *Citrus aurantium* var. *senensis* is not so useful.) A luxury oil used mainly for its aroma, it is a very effective anti-depressant. Belonging to the Rutaceae family, it is distilled mostly in

Mediterranean countries. Its pale yellow oil is indispensible in the making of good quality eau-de-colognes, and orange flower water is a by-product of distillation. The best oils come from France and Tunisia, and although expensive it is economical in use; it has a tenacious aroma. Not to be confused with orange blossom oil, which is an absolute from the same flowers, extracted by using a solvent; this has a headier and sweeter aroma and contains different constituents which are not soluble in steam.

Circulation: haemorrhoids, high blood pressure, poor circulation, varicose veins
Digestive: chronic diarrhoea (due to stress), sluggish liver
Menstrual: PMS
Nervous: agitation, anxiety, depression, fear, insomnia, irritability
Skin: all types, especially dry, broken capillaries, mature, sensitive

### Nutmeg *(Myristica fragrans)*

*Blends well with:*
clove
juniper
rosemary
sage

A member of the Myristicaceae family, the seeds of the nutmeg tree are distilled to give us essential oil of nutmeg. The seed itself is very interesting in that the outer lace-like covering, mace, was once regarded as more important than the nutmeg, which was thrown away.

Digestive: abdominal cramp, chronic diarrhoea, flatulence, loss of appetite, sluggish digestion
Head: bad breath, toothache
Menstrual: scanty periods
Muscular: aches and pains, muscular pain, rheumatism, sprains
Nervous: debility, neuralgia
Special: facilitates delivery in childbirth

*Note:* Nutmeg is neurotoxic when used incorrectly and should be used with care and advice, as it is hallucinogenic in overdose.

## Origanum *(Origanum heracleoticum)*

*Blends well with:*
bergamot
black pepper
juniper

This plant (another Lamiate), is often referred to as wild marjoram, and the flowering tops and leaves are used in the distillation process. Botanically, all the origanums are difficult to sort out and no-one is quite sure how they should be classified.

Digestive: infections of the digestive tract
Excretory: infections of the urinary tract
Nervous: debility (tonic)
Respiratory: infections of the respiratory tract
Skin: lice, parasites
Special: low immune system

*Note:* like savory and phenolic thymes, origanum is a powerful oil and needs care or advice with use.

## Patchouli *(Pogostemon patchouli)*

*Blends well with:*
bergamot
geranium
lavender
myrrh
neroli
pine needle
rose otto

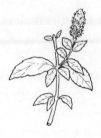

Surprisingly enough, patchouli belongs to the *Lamiate* family. The oil is obtained from young leaves, which are cut whenever five are growing on one stem at any one time, and dried before being steam distilled. No oil is present in the older leaves. Patchouli is interesting in that small quantities will uplift but larger doses sedate. Probably originating in the Philippine Islands, the main supply now comes from Indonesia, and is mostly distilled in Singapore.

Circulatory: haemorrhoids, varicose veins
Digestive: gastro-enteritis
Skin: acne, allergies, cellulite (decongestant), eczema, heals chapped and cracked skin, inflammation, regenerative, scar tissue
Special: low immune system

**Rose Otto** *(Rosa damascena; R. centifolia)*

*Blends well with:*
bergamot
clary-sage
geranium
jasmine
patchouli
sandalwood
and many more

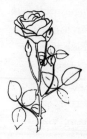

This illustrious oil flower is used to produce a distilled oil and an absolute. Bulgarian roses *(Rosa damascena)* are reputed to give the best distilled oil (rose otto), and Morocco is the largest producer of rose oils from *Rosa centifolia*. The distilled oil is the best for therapeutic use. In France the production of rose otto is very small, most of the rose oil being produced there being rose absolute. Rose oil is sometimes produced as a by-product from the making of rose water, when the essential oil floats on the top. Like melissa and neroli, although expensive, very little is needed, and it should be used where the aroma is of importance. Having extremely low toxicity (yet being very powerful), rose otto is a safe choice for children.

Head: mouth ulcers
Menstrual: frigidity, irregular menstruation
Muscular: sprains
Nervous: debility, depression
Respiratory: asthma, bronchitis
Skin: antiseptic, blotchy, chapped or cracked, inflamed, mature, sensitive, wounds

## Sandalwood *(Santalum album)*

*Blends well with:*
benzoin
black pepper
cypress
frankincense
neroli
ylang-ylang

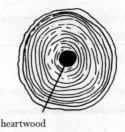

heartwood

Sandalwood belongs to a family called Santalaceae and the best essential oils come from trees grown in the area which used to be called Mysore, in East India. Production is carefully controlled and regulated by the government because the trees take so long to mature, reaching a height of 60–65ft. The evergreen trees are not cut down until fully mature and showing signs of dying. The oil is mainly in the heartwood at the centre of the tree (not in the bark) and the roots. The heartwood takes 30 years to become 3 inches (7cm) in diameter, and the oil is obtained by steam distillation. The best trees are used for wood for cabinet making, the off-cuts and roots being distilled. Next to rose, sandalwood is the most precious in the history of perfume.

Circulatory: haemorrhoids, varicose veins
Digestive: diarrhoea, heartburn, nausea (in pregnancy)
Excretory: cystitis, diuretic, urinary tract infections
Nervous: neuralgia, sciatica, tension
Respiratory: bronchitis, 'flu, hiccups
Skin: acne, chapped and cracked, dry, eczema (dry), sunburn (soothing)

**Ylang-Ylang** *(Cananga odorata)*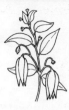

*Blends well with most oils, especially:*
jasmine
sandalwood

Obtained by distillation from the flowers (the name 'ylang-ylang', from the Annonaceae family, means 'flower of flowers'). The best plants are grown in the Philippines and Reunion. In Manila the tree blossoms all the year round, although the best flowers for oil are picked in May and June only, early in the morning. Ylang-ylang is much used in high-class perfumery, and often called the poor man's jasmine. Many different qualities of oil are available and oil from Javanese trees of the same name is decidedly inferior, probably due to climatic and soil conditions. Dry soil, high elevation, shade from olive trees and *spring* rain give a much superior oil than that from rich moist soil at low levels. It can take up to 18, or even 24 hours to distil ylang-ylang and the oil is collected in fractions during this time, yielding several incomplete portions of the oil. The lightest molecules to vaporize make up extra and superior grades, followed by grades 1, 2 and 3. The complete oil would be the best for aromatherapy (even though it does not have the best aroma), but it is not easy to obtain an unadulterated complete oil of ylang-ylang as the extra and superior grades are in great demand by the perfume industry, the lower grades 2 and 3 especially being less useful as their solubility in alcohol is less and the aroma not so exotic.

Circulation: high blood pressure
Digestive: diabetes, gastro-enteritis, intestinal infections
Head: thinning hair (scalp tonic)
Menstrual: frigidity
Nervous: agitation, insomnia, tension (sedative)

# chapter twelve

# THERAPEUTIC INDEX

| Problem | Top Notes | Middle Notes | Base Notes |
|---|---|---|---|
| **Circulation** | | | |
| anaemia | lemon, phenolic thyme | | |
| chilblains | lemon | lavender | |
| haemorrhoids (piles) | cajuput, clary sage, niaouli, tea tree | cypress, geranium, sandalwood | neroli, patchouli, |
| high blood pressure | lemon, niaouli | lavender, marjoram, melissa, rosemary (low dose) | neroli, ylang-ylang |
| low blood pressure | basil, phenolic thyme, sage | hyssop, peppermint, pine, rosemary (high dose), savory | clove |
| poor circulation | lemon, orange, phenolic thyme, sage | black pepper, cypress, neroli, rosemary | benzoin, ginger, |
| sluggish lymph | sage | geranium, pine, rosemary | cedarwood |
| varicose veins | cajuput, clary sage, lemon, niaouli, sage, tea tree | cypress, geranium, sandalwood | neroli, patchouli, |
| **Digestive** | | | |
| colic | bergamot, cajuput | aniseed, chamomile (R), geranium, hyssop, lavender, marjoram, peppermint, savory | |

| Problem | Top Notes | Middle Notes | Base Notes |
|---|---|---|---|
| colitis, enteritis | lemongrass, niaouli, tea tree (viral), thyme (sweet) | fennel, geranium, peppermint, rosemary, savory | neroli |
| constipation | orange | fennel, hyssop (mild) rosemary | ginger |
| diabetes | lemon, sweet thyme | geranium, juniper, pine, rosemary | neroli, ylang-ylang |
| diarrhoea | lemon, niaouli, sage | chamomile (R), geranium, marjoram, rosemary, savory | clove, ginger, neroli (chronic) nutmeg, sandalwood |
| flatulence | basil, bergamot, caraway, coriander, lemon, phenolic thyme, sage | aniseed, chamomile (Roman), fennel, hyssop, lavender, marjoram, peppermint, rosemary, savory | clove, ginger, myrrh, nutmeg |
| gall stones | lemon, niaouli | hyssop, peppermint, pine, rosemary | |
| gastric spasm | caraway, orange | chamomile (German), marjoram, melissa, peppermint, savory | clove |
| gastro-enteritis | basil, cajuput, coriander, lemon, lemongrass, niaouli, sweet thyme, tea tree | chamomile (G), fennel, geranium, lavandin, lavender, peppermint, rosemary, savory | clove, origanum, patchouli, ylang-ylang |

| Problem | Top Notes | Middle Notes | Base Notes |
|---|---|---|---|
| heartburn | orange | peppermint | sandalwood |
| indigestion (dyspepsia) | basil, bergamot, caraway, coriander, niaouli, orange, sage | aniseed (nervous), black pepper, chamomile (R), fennel, hyssop, lavender, marjoram, melissa, peppermint, rosemary | clove, ginger (painful) |
| liver (sluggish) | sage, sweet thyme | black pepper, chamomile (M, geranium, melissa, peppermint, rosemary | |
| loss of appetite | bergamot, caraway, lemon, sage | aniseed, chamomile (R), fennel, hyssop, juniper, | ginger, myrrh, nutmeg, |
| nausea | lemon | chamomile (G), fennel, lavender, melissa (morning sickness), peppermint | ginger, sandalwood (in pregnancy) |
| sluggish digestion | basil, coriander, lemongrass, phenolic thyme, sage | black pepper, hyssop, savory | ginger, nutmeg |
| stomach pains | bergamot, lemon | chamomile, fennel, lavender, melissa (cramp), peppermint pine, rosemary, savory | nutmeg |

| Problem | Top Notes | Middle Notes | Base Notes |
|---|---|---|---|
| stomach ulcers | lemon | lavender, peppermint, pine, rosemary, savory chamomile (G), geranium, | |
| travel sickness | basil | peppermint | |
| vomiting | lemon | aniseed (nervous), fennel, peppermint (nervous) | |
| **Excretory** | | | |
| bedwetting | | cypress, rosemary | |
| cystitis | cajuput, coriander, eucalyptus, niaouli, sweet and phenolic thyme | chamomile (M), fennel, hyssop, juniper, lavender, peppermint, pine, rosemary, savory | cedarwood, clove, sandalwood |
| diuretic | eucalyptus, lemon, sage, sweet thyme | aniseed, cypress, fennel, geranium (mild), hyssop, juniper, rosemary | sandalwood |
| fluid retention | lemon, sage | cypress, fennel, geranium, juniper, rosemary | cedarwood, sandalwood, patchouli |
| infections | niaouli, sweet thyme | black pepper, fennel, pine | myrrh, origanum, sandalwood |

| Problem | Top Notes | Middle Notes | Base Notes |
|---|---|---|---|
| kidneys (general) | eucalyptus, lemon | geranium, juniper, pine | cedarwood, sandalwood |
| stones | lemon | fennel, geranium, hyssop, juniper | |
| **Head (and Scalp)** | | | |
| alopecia (hair loss) | caraway, clary-sage, sage, thyme (phenolic) | rosemary | cedarwood, ylang-ylang |
| bad breath | | peppermint, rosemary | clove, nutmeg |
| colds | basil, cajuput, eucalyptus, lemon, niaouli, phenolic and sweet thyme | black pepper, hyssop, marjoram peppermint, pine, rosemary | benzoin |
| dandruff | | rosemary | cedarwood |
| earache | basil, cajuput (inflammation), sweet thyme | lavender, rosemary | |
| hay fever | caraway | hyssop | rose otto |
| headaches and migraines | lemon, eucalyptus (congestive) | aniseed, black pepper (due to head cold), chamomile (R), lavandin (chronic), lavender, marjoram, melissa, peppermint (digestive), rosemary | |
| laryngitis | cajuput, eucalyptus, sage, | sweet thyme, black pepper, peppermint | myrrh |

| Problem | Top Notes | Middle Notes | Base Notes |
|---|---|---|---|
| lice | thyme (phenolic) | | origanum |
| mouth ulcers | lemon, orange, sage, tea tree | rosemary geranium | myrrh, rose |
| mouthwash (gum strengthener) | lemon, sage, tea tree | chamomile (R), fennel | myrrh |
| nose bleed | lemon | cypress | |
| seborrhoea (greasy) | lemon | juniper | cedarwood |
| sinusitis | basil, cajuput, eucalyptus, lemon, niaouli, sage, sweet and phenolic thyme, tea tree | hyssop, lavender, marjoram, peppermint, pine, rosemary | clove |
| sore throat | bergamot, eucalyptus, lemon, niaouli, phenolic and sweet thyme, sage, tea tree | geranium, lavandin, lavender, savory | ginger, sandalwood |
| teething | | chamomile (R) | |
| tonsillitis | bergamot, sweet thyme | geranium, savory | |
| toothache | cajuput, sage | black pepper, chamomile (R), marjoram | clove, ginger, nutmeg |
| vertigo (dizziness) | basil, caraway, lemongrass, orange | aniseed, marjoram, melissa peppermint, rosemary | |

| Problem | Top Notes | Middle Notes | Base Notes |
|---|---|---|---|
| **Menstrual** | | | |
| irregularity | basil, clary-sage, niaouli, sage | chamomile (R & G), fennel, hyssop, lavender, melissa, peppermint (ovarian stimulant) | rose otto |
| lack of periods | clary-sage, niaouli, sage | anised, chamomile (R & G), fennel, melissa, rosemary | |
| leucorrhoea | bergamot | geranium, hyssop, lavender | myrrh |
| menopause | clary-sage, sage | anised, chamomile (R), fennel, peppermint (hot flushes) | |
| ovary problems | sage | cypress, fennel, peppermint | |
| painful | cajuput, clary-sage, sage | anised, chamomile (R & G), fennel, geranium, melissa, pine, rosemary | jasmine |
| PMS | clary-sage, tea-tree | anised, chamomile (G), fennel, geranium, hyssop, lavender, melissa | neroli |
| scanty | sage | hyssop, lavender, melissa, peppermint, rosemary | nutmeg |

| Problem | Top Notes | Middle Notes | Base Notes |
|---|---|---|---|
| **Muscular** | | | |
| aches and pains | cajuput, coriander, eucalyptus, sage, sweet thyme | aniseed, black pepper, chamomile (Roman, German and Moroccan), juniper, lavandin, lavender, marjoram, rosemary | clove, frankincense, ginger, nutmeg, origanum |
| arthritis | basil, cajuput, coriander, eucalyptus, lemon, niaouli, sage, sweet thyme | aniseed, chamomile (Roman, German and Moroccan), juniper, geranium, lavender, marjoram, pine, savory | benzoin, clove |
| cramp, spasm | basil | cypress, geranium, lavender, marjoram, rosemary | |
| rheumatism | cajuput, coriander, eucalyptus, lemon, niaouli, sage, phenolic and sweet thyme | aniseed, chamomile (R, G & M), geranium, hyssop, juniper, lavandin, lavender, marjoram, pine, rosemary, savory | clove, frankincense, ginger, nutmeg, origanum |
| sprains | eucalyptus | hyssop, lavender, marjoram, rosemary | nutmeg, rose otto |
| lack of tone | lemongrass | black pepper | |

| Problem | Top Notes | Middle Notes | Base Notes |
|---|---|---|---|
| **Nervous** | | | |
| agitation (excitability, tantrums) | bergamot | cypress, lavender, geranium, marjoram, melissa, rosemary | neroli, nutmeg, ylang-ylang |
| anxiety (tension) | basil, bergamot, clary-sage, orange, phenolic and sweet thyme | chamomile (R), geranium, lavender, marjoram, melissa | frankincense, neroli, rose otto ylang-ylang |
| apathy | coriander, petitgrain | geranium, melissa, peppermint | jasmine, neroli |
| debility (run down) | basil, clary-sage, coriander, sage, thyme (phenolic and sweet) | chamomile (M), cypress, geranium, juniper, lavandin, lavender, marjoram, peppermint, pine, rosemary, savory | benzoin, clove, jasmine nutmeg, origanum, rose otto |
| depression | basil, bergamot, clary-sage, thyme (phenolic and sweet) tea tree | chamomile (R & M), geranium, lavender, savory | frankincense, jasmine, neroli, patchouli, rose otto, sandalwood |
| fatigue (mental) | basil, coriander, thyme (phenolic and sweet) | rosemary, savory | clove |
| fatigue (general – nerve tonic) | basil, coriander, sage thyme (sweet) | geranium, juniper, melissa, pine, rosemary (fainting) | clove, ginger, origanum |

| Problem | Top Notes | Middle Notes | Base Notes |
|---------|-----------|--------------|------------|
| insomnia | basil, lemon, orange, petitgrain, thyme (sweet) | chamomile (R), juniper, lavender, marjoram, melissa | neroli, sandalwood, ylang-ylang |
| irritability | petitgrain | chamomile (R), cypress, lavender, marjoram, melissa | neroli, rose otto |
| neuralgia | cajuput, eucalyptus | chamomile (Roman), geranium, peppermint, rosemary | clove, nutmeg, sandalwood |
| palpitations | lemongrass, orange | aniseed, fennel, lavender, marjoram, melissa, rosemary | |
| vertigo (dizziness) | caraway, lemongrass, orange | aniseed, marjoram, melissa, peppermint, rosemary | |
| **Respiratory** asthma | cajuput, eucalyptus, lemon sage, phenolic and sweet thyme | aniseed, hyssop, lavender, marjoram, peppermint, pine, rosemary, savory | benzoin, clove, frankincense, rose otto |
| bronchitis | cajuput (chronic), caraway, eucalyptus, lemon, niaouli, sage, tea tree, phenolic and sweet thyme | aniseed, black pepper, cypress, hyssop, lavandin, lavender marjoram, peppermint, pine, rosemary, savory | benzoin, cedarwood, clove, frankincense, ginger (chronic), myrrh, neroli, rose otto, sandalwood |

| Problem | Top Notes | Middle Notes | Base Notes |
|---------|-----------|--------------|------------|
| catarrh | eucalyptus, lemon, niaouli | aniseed, black pepper, hyssop lavender, marjoram, savory | benzoin, cedarwood, frankincense, myrrh |
| coughs | cajuput, eucalyptus, niaouli, thyme (phenolic and sweet) | aniseed, black pepper, cypress (spasmodic), hyssop, lavandin, lavender, marjoram pine, rosemary, savory | benzoin, cedarwood, cinnamon, origanum |
| 'flu | cajuput, eucalyptus, lemon, sage, phenolic and sweet thyme | cypress, hyssop, lavender, pine, rosemary | benzoin, myrrh, sandalwood |
| **Skin** | | | |
| acne | lemongrass, petitgrain, tea tree, phenolic and sweet thyme | chamomile (M), geranium, juniper, lavandin, lavender | cedarwood, clove (infected), patchouli, sandalwood |
| allergy prone and sensitive | | chamomile (R) | neroli, patchouli, rose otto |
| animal bites | sage | lavender | |
| boils and abcesses | lemon, niaouli, tea tree, phenolic and sweet thyme | chamomile (R & M), lavender, savory | clove, myrrh |
| broken capillaries | lemon | cypress, peppermint | neroli, rose otto |
| bruises | | cypress, hyssop, lavender, marjoram, rosemary | |
| burns | | chamomile (R), geranium, lavender, rosemary | benzoin |

| Problem | Top Notes | Middle Notes | Base Notes |
|---|---|---|---|
| cellulite | sage, thyme (sweet) | fennel, juniper, rosemary | cedarwood, origanum, patchouli |
| chapped and cracked | | chamomile (R), geranium | benzoin, patchouli, rose otto, sandalwood |
| congested | basil, lemon, sage | geranium, rosemary | |
| dermatitis | sage, sweet thyme | chamomile (M), geranium, hyssop, juniper, lavender | benzoin |
| dry | petitgrain | chamomile, lavender | benzoin, jasmine, neroli, rose otto, sandalwood |
| eczema (general) | sage, thyme (sweet) | chamomile (R, G & M) geranium, hyssop, peppermint lavender | cedarwood |
| (dry) | basil | lavender | |
| (weeping) | bergamot | juniper | |
| fungal infections (i.e. athlete's foot) | clary-sage, niaouli | geranium, lavandin lavender | benzoin, patchouli, sandalwood |
| herpes simplex I (cold sores) | bergamot, eucalyptus, lemon | lavender, melissa, peppermint, savory | cedarwood, patchouli |

| Problem | Top Notes | Middle Notes | Base Notes |
|---|---|---|---|
| inflamed | clary-sage | chamomile (R & G), geranium, lavender, peppermint, pine lavender, melissa (bee), savory | frankincense, myrrh, patchouli, rose otto, sandalwood |
| insect bites and stings | basil (wasp), lemon, niaouli, sage, tea tree, thyme (sweet) | | |
| insect repellent | basil, cajuput, eucalyptus, lemongrass | geranium | cedarwood, clove (mosquitoes) |
| irritable (itchy) | | chamomile (R), lavender, peppermint (less than 1% i.e. 5 drops in 50ml) | benzoin, cedarwood, neroli, sandalwood |
| mature (rejuvenating: wrinkles) | clary-sage, lemon, niaouli, orange | fennel, lavender, melissa | benzoin, frankincense, myrrh, neroli, rose otto patchouli |
| oedema | lemon, petitgrain | fennel, geranium, juniper | |
| oily (open pores) | lemon, lemongrass, orange, petitgrain | cypress, geranium, juniper, lavandin, lavender | cedarwood |
| poor tone | orange, lemongrass, niaouli, sage | geranium, rosemary | frankincense |
| psoriasis | bergamot, cajuput, niaouli, thyme (sweet) | lavender | benzoin |

| Problem | Top Notes | Middle Notes | Base Notes |
|---|---|---|---|
| regenerating | | lavender | frankincense, myrrh, neroli, patchouli |
| scars | | | frankincense, patchouli |
| shingles | sage, sweet thyme | hyssop, lavender | |
| stretch marks (also see 'poor tone' above) | | geranium, melissa lavender, geranium | frankincense, myrrh |
| sunburn | | lavender, peppermint (no more than 2 drops in 10ml) | sandalwood |
| super sensitive | | chamomile (R) | neroli, rose otto |
| sweating (perspiration) | clary-sage, sage | cypress, peppermint, pine (feet) | |
| ulcers | eucalyptus, niaouli | chamomile (G), juniper, geranium, lavender (varicose) | clove, frankincense, myrrh |
| wounds | eucalyptus, niaouli, tea tree (infected), thyme (phenolic) (infected) | chamomile (R & G), geranium, hyssop, juniper, lavandin, lavender, rosemary, savory | benzoin, clove, cedarwood, frankincense, myrrh, patchouli, rose otto |

| Problem | Top Notes | Middle Notes | Base Notes |
|---|---|---|---|
| **Special** | | | |
| breastfeeding problems | | | |
| (lack of milk) | | aniseed, fennel | jasmine |
| (too much milk) | | peppermint | |
| candida | eucalyptus, sage, tea tree, thyme (sweet) | geranium, lavandin, lavender, rosemary, savory | |
| gout | basil, cajuput, lemon | chamomile (R), fennel, juniper, pine, rosemary | benzoin |
| hormone like | cajuput, clary-sage, niaouli, sage | chamomile (G), fennel, juniper, lavender, marjoram, melissa, peppermint, pine, rosemary | myrrh |
| labour (facilities delivery in childbirth) | sage, sweet thyme | aniseed, peppermint | clove (long labour), nutmeg |
| low immune system | lemon, niaouli, tea tree, sweet thyme | savory | clove, frankincense, origanum, patchouli |
| warts and veruccas | lemon, sweet thyme | | |
| loss of memory (mental stimulant) | | peppermint | clove |
| sciatica | phenolic thyme | aniseed | sandalwood |

# chapter thirteen

It is always exciting and stimulating to read about successful case histories, but at the same time it must be remembered that for every ten spectacular cases there are ten with only mediocre results and possibly one or two on whom very little change is noticed. These are the people who probably need another form of natural treatment as back up, such as acupuncture, reflexology, diet or naturopathy. Also, if *only* the symptoms are being treated, or if it is not clear what is *causing* the symptoms and therefore the wrong choice of oil is made, then the results cannot be expected to be miraculous. Don't give up, simply try a different mix of essential oils.

I have one case history myself of just such a happening. The daughter of a friend of mine was having problems with recurring eczema and wanted to try a natural remedy. I mixed her an eczema cream and she was delighted with the results. She has been clear enough only to need her second pot twelve months later. A few weeks later she rang me to ask if I could mix something for her boyfriend who had a 'sort of prickly heat' rash for a few weeks and the irritation was getting him down. So I mixed him an oil containing peppermint and sandalwood ... I didn't see Hazel for a while but when I did she said it hadn't done a lot for his rash. It did lessen the irritation, but it wasn't clearing up. After further conversation (not having ever seen him, by the way!) I came to the conclusion that it may be a type of contact dermatitis, and suggested that I see him before mixing any further oils. After trying a lotion for dermatitis, and sourcing the cause of the irritation (a change in his mother's washing powder!) I am happy to say his problem cleared up.

A client of mine, Mrs F. of Hinckley, whom I met when giving a talk on aromatherapy at a ladies night did not have success on my first attempt to clear up the blotchy, dry skin on her face. I first of all gave her the moisturizer from my Professional range for a dry skin, and after four days her skin was no better, but even drier than before! (I must add here that she had been using a mineral oil based moisturizer, which tends to draw moisture from below your skin surface as well as the air, in order to keep the surface moist, so without that her skin was extra dry.) She came to the clinic where I gave her a face mask to stimulate blood circulation, and I asked her to take her moisture cream into work and apply it every two hours. After a week she rang me up to say that it was back to 'normal' and no longer extra dry but it was still blotchy and as dry as when I first met her. Not many ladies would have persevered as Susan did, and I am very grateful to her for that, as I really wanted to get to the bottom of it. She came again to the clinic, where my husband, who is a trichologist (and covered diseases of the skin in his training) asked if there was any history of eczema, asthma or hay fever in her family. 'Yes' was the answer – though she herself had no symptoms – whereupon Len suggested I mix a moisture cream containing oils for training eczema. This I did, and a delighted Mrs F. came into see me two weeks later, with a lovely clear and soft skin – no blotches or dry patches. Needless to say she has been using this special moisture cream ever since.

I am really grateful for her perseverance; many would have just assumed themselves allergic to this new product and gone back to their other one, without contacting me and giving me a chance to try something else. The *only* difference between the first moisture cream she tried and the second was in the essential oils I used. Now, whenever I meet anyone with a problem like Mrs F.'s, I always ask about the eczema, asthma or hay fever link, and so far I have had great success. I call it my 'Special E' cream (the 'E' does not stand for vitamin E, but for the fact that essential oils for eczema are in it). Mrs F. uses the normal cleanser for dry skin.

Mrs U., also of Hinckley, had a hip replacement nearly four years ago. This didn't 'take' and after many complications and a lot of pain she has had the replacement removed. The skin on her leg is very dry since the operation, so she uses my after bath lotion which keeps her skin from flaking. The arthritis oil I mixed for her has helped the pain in her hands and shoulders considerably, and a few weeks ago I mixed her an oil for bruises as the slightest knock comes up in a bruise. It is actually an oil to prevent stretch marks and I have had success with stretch marks *after* pregnancy with this particular mix of essential oils. I first prepared the oil for someone who didn't take care *during* pregnancy to prevent stretch marks appearing in the first place.

J., one of my staff, used my anti-stretch mark oil all during her first pregnancy and because she was so delighted recommended it to K., another girl on my staff who became pregnant. M., who tested the stretch mark oil on her six year old stretch marks, also tested an oil I made for cellulite and fluid retention, with results that were sufficient for her husband to notice the difference on her thighs.

Mrs L. from Hinckley is using this same oil for fluid retention in her ankles. She was having to take two water tablets a day and the continual visits to the toilet were making her feel weak and miserable. After one week of massaging my oil into her lower legs and feet (in an upward direction only), her ankles had gone down about one inch (2½cm) in circumference. She told her doctor, because she was so delighted (he is my doctor too!) and he laughed, saying 'Ah, yes, Shirley and her ideas – it won't do you any harm, anyway!' Mrs L. is now only taking *one* water tablet a day and her ankles have stayed less swollen.

A client of mine has a young 8-year-old with eczema. Caroline puts the problem skin lotion on herself, and whenever the eczema appears it will clear up when she uses her special lotion. Her mother has now asked me to mix something for her own lack of facial muscle tone. A few weeks ago she came to my salon for a course of electrical facial treatments to rejuvenate tired and dry skins. I recommended using the creams accompanying the treatment at home between each visit, which she did, and liked them very much. Unfortunately they proved too expensive to keep up, so I suggested she try my own range, with essential oils to treat dry and lined skin. She swears her skin is even better than before and I must admit that the Professional night cream has done wonders for her neck.

Mrs F. is a client who suffers from psoriasis. This is a difficult problem to treat as it returns from time to time. Mrs F. started using my skin problem lotion about two years ago and finds that with regular daily use she never has a severe breakout like she used to have.

P, who is now 26, had a nervous rash four years ago which left her with severe irritation all over her body in cold weather. A mixture of sandalwood and peppermint in the right proportions was a great help to her at these times, keeping the irritation at bay. As soon as her nervous problem was resolved, the 'symptoms' (i.e. the rash) disappeared altogether and she no longer needed the oils. When she was better, we then tackled her period problems. She did not begin to menstruate until she was 16, and then very spasmodically, sometimes going for as long as seven months without a period. She also had a weight problem from about the same age and used to fast for three or four days at a time, drinking only liquids. She did this because if she exceeded 500 calories a day she put on weight! Then she would get fed up and nibble one or two biscuits with her coffee on a 'fasting' day, and of course her weight was never stable. When she was on vacation from college, we decided to tackle the periods with essential oils. I mixed her an oil containing rose otto, Roman chamomile and true melissa to massage on her tummy, and a neat essential oil mix for her bath, every other day. Within a week she had a period, and we continued with the treatment. Six weeks later she had another period and they are now coming every four or five weeks without using the oils. *But*, one of the biggest benefits was that after the periods began to come regularly she shed her surplus weight, now eats normally (but eats no butter, though a lot of bran and fibre) and is a size 12, much to her delight!

Cramp is another problem which is very easily helped with essential oils. I haven't yet had a failure with it. My first success was Mrs P. of Sharnford, who suffered badly with cramp during the night. I mixed her an oil to massage into her left foot and calf each night for the first week and once a week thereafter, and a bath oil to put into her bath once a week. She has never had cramp since and that was two and a half years ago. When she went to Australia to live with her daughter she took a year's supply with her!

B. is a client of mine who also acts as a model for me when I am teaching aromatherapy to other people on my courses. She had severe cramp pains in the toes of her left foot. I gave her 'a magic little bottle of oils' (in her own words) 'and even after two nights the pain had almost disappeared. At the first sign of recurrence of pain I only have to use it for one night and it disappears.'

My friend from Earl Shilton also suffered from cramp, but no longer does. Her husband used the same oil for his sprained knee and fortunately the sweet marjoram in her oil was the essential oil for sprains too – though neither knew that at the time he used it! I have since mixed a successful oil for her mother-in-law for rheumatism, and an insect repellent for her daughter, who went to Africa this year on holiday! Last year, she asked me if I could do anything for her sinuses – she was considering an operation, but prefered to try aromatherapy first, just in case it might help. In her own words:

'I have suffered from sinusitis for several years, with frequent severe attacks, especially during the winter. My face was often swollen and painful along the cheek bone, and I suffered with headaches. One winter the condition was so persistent I asked Shirley if she could help. She gave me an oil for putting in the bath and an oil for massaging into the face, with detailed instructions about the pressures to do along the area of the sinus blockage.

'Initially I used the bath oil two or three times a week, now only once a week. The massage oil was used initially every night. After four weeks I had considerable relief from the condition. Shirley then suggested that instead of using her normal night cream with the oils in for skin rejuvenation, I should use one with oils in for sinus problems. I use this every night, as I did the other night cream, and whenever I get a cold I use the massage oil with my pressures.

'Result – the sinus condition is greatly improved, even with a cold; it seems able to prevent mucus congestion, and I haven't had a severe attack ever since.'

Mr C., a patient of my husband, complained of scalp eruptions and intense irritation. Having tried one of his own trichology lotions on Mr C. without total success, Len asked me if I could suggest one of my oils. I made up a base cream with the eczema oils in it for him to try (pure guess work!) and there was an instant improvement. One 100g pot was sufficient to return his scalp to normal, and he uses Len's special shampoo to keep it clear.

Mrs J. came to see Len with similar eruptions on her face and many tiny lumps under the skin surface. Any skin product irritated the condition, so Len asked me if I could mix her a face moisturizer for use after washing, and Mrs J. still uses 'Special E Cream' as her daily moisturizer. Again it was the eczema oils which brought success.

Hair loss is a difficult condition to treat, but I have found that regular *correct* massage definitely prevents further thinning, and in quite a number of cases actually revives hair follicles which have lost the ability to produce hair. To do the massage, 'glue' your fingers to the scalp and move the scalp over the bone for a few seconds. Move to a different place and repeat. This massage is preceded by the application of carrier oil – containing rosemary and cedarwood – sparingly along the scalp in rows every half inch and spread evenly by moving your fingers lightly backwards and forwards all over the scalp. The texture of the hair improves and thickening is noticeable after six to eight months of *regular* daily use. Cases are too numerous to mention, but at least eight women and five men have benefited from this treatment and names can be supplied on request.

The following case histories, which have been sent to me by practising aromatherapists and reflexologists whom I have trained, have not been re-written.

From Mrs Teresa Silva:

> I would inform you that Miss P. was involved in a nasty car accident about five years ago. Her back and neck got knocked about over this accident. For two years she has been unable to resume her work, and lead a normal life. However for the past three years she has been coping, although unable to sleep through one night without interruption, due to pain in her neck.
>
> Another complaint was the lack of punctuality over her period cycle, and the swelling over her tummy. She also suffers considerably from constipation.
>
> On the 25th August, I gave her my first treatment using the following oils: melissa, marjoram, lavender, juniper.
>
> On the 26th August, she telephoned me at 10 a.m. excitedly to inform me that for the first time in a very long period she had slept right through the night. Moreover, her period was right on time, and also there was no constipation.
>
> On the 3rd September (second treatment) she is still sleeping normally, the pain on her back has subsided, and is now much more bearable, although there is still some tenderness in her tummy.

I shall endeavour to enquire further from her prior to seeing you on the 20th.

From Keith and Terry Clarke:

In our clinic, an experiment combining a course of aromatherapy in conjunction with acupuncture treatments, in cases of either severe arthritis or stress, has proved to be very successful. So much so, that our clients have returned after completion of treatments, requesting aromatherapy for the pure enjoyment of it. The following case-histories were particularly rewarding:

*Case 'A'* paid us a visit in May/June requesting acupuncture treatment for severe arthritis in the bottom of her spine, also in her hips. Her trouble had begun in December/January, since when she had been unable to walk any distance without pain, had difficulty in getting in and out of a chair, and was unable to sleep. Acupuncture was prescribed twice weekly for the first month, during which time the condition improved enough for an aromatherapy course to be introduced. The oils to be used were of lavender, benzoin and rosemary. Both the acupuncture and the aromatherapy treatments were given at the rate of one per week for approximately three weeks, after which, both treatments were gradually reduced to once per month – alternating fortnightly. The lady in question by the month of November was 90 per cent free from her pain.

*Case 'B'* came to us in late August with severe pain resulting from an old disc problem. She had requested acupuncture treatment which of course was agreed upon. But we also suggested that it should be combined with a course of aromatherapy and this was also arranged – the oils used were of rosemary, benzoin, lavender. Both treatments were given at intervals of approximately ten days, and our client gradually improved. By mid-October she had returned to work and now only calls upon us occasionally.

*Case 'C'* who had suffered severe neurosis for some considerable period of time, contacted us for acupuncture treatment in July to help her condition. After discussing her problem at great length, it was agreed that the treatment would be carried out in the surroundings of her own home. It was necessary to treat her twice weekly for approximately three weeks before introducing a course of aromatherapy, again in conjunction with the acupuncture. The oils used were of chamomile, juniper, marjoram, lavender. The initial treatments were at intervals of approximately five or six days. After her second aromatherapy, our client became much more able to relax, and both the aromatherapy and acupuncture treatments were gradually reduced to fortnightly visits. Although still undergoing treatments – this is now November and our client is able to travel to our clinic for a monthly visit. This is, of course, nearing the completion of all her treatments.

From Doreen Bader:

Mr T. was experiencing general tension, scalp tight, circulation poor in feet, indigestion problems. I used ylang-ylang and rosemary for his face; lavender, bergamot and juniper for the body. I massaged Mr T. once a week for five consecutive weeks and after that period (in fact well before) he was sleeping far better and relaxing and in fact he was able to leave off taking sleeping tablets and Valium.

Mrs B. had very bad rheumatism in the feet and hands. I did massage on these areas over a four week period and she was able to move her toes (which before she was unable to do) and her hands were more flexible and less painful. I used for the massage sage, rosemary and lavender.

Ms T. had very badly swollen legs and ankles, and had had treatment at the local hospital – physiotherapy – which had not helped at all. I have been massaging this lady's legs and ankles twice a week over a four week period and even after the first two sessions there was a noticeable reduction in the swellings. She is now delighted to be able to see her ankle bones and her legs are the normal size too (there were unsightly bumps before which have now gone down). I used for this lady sage, rosemary and lavender.

Mrs B. had a very painful knee and I used both aromatherapy massage and Swiss Reflex Therapy on the knee reflex on her feet to help. This alleviated the pain.

Ms W. had pain around the sciatic nerve and I massaged her feet around this area, again using SRT, (also massage part of the leg) and she has not had a recurrence!

From Siobhann O'Donovan:

Mrs B. had kidney problems, tension and cough. When doing the reflex assessment on the feet, the kidney was quite painful; this was pointed out to the client, which confirmed her suspicions that she did in fact have a weak kidney. This client also suffered from bronchitis. When Mrs B. returned home, after the massage treatment using eucalyptus and lavender, she slept for a good deal of the afternoon which is quite out of character. When she awoke she found that her breathing was not as tight as it had been in the past, and the niggling pain from her kidney had gone.

*Mrs M.*: bronchitis and poor circulation
*Treatment:* eucalyptus, juniper.
When doing thumb pressure down the spine this client coughed continuously and I could feel all the nodules dispersing. A few hours after leaving the salon the client 'phoned to say that she had been able to dislodge all the mucus from her chest which then allowed her to breathe normally again.

*Mrs H.*: cellulite, poor circulation
*Treatment:* juniper.
This client is only having a leg massage as she is very embarrassed about the cellulite in her thighs. She is a very independent lady by nature and felt quite disgusted with herself for allowing them to reach this condition and not be able to treat them herself. She then sought the help of aromatherapy and I am working on the drainage principle. After about three weeks a visible difference was noticed which gave the client the confidence and will power to continue the treatment, therefore giving her confidence in herself. Now, after ten weeks, there is a great improvement in the condition of her thighs.

From Janice Benham:

Miss C., 18 years old. Backache that had lasted approximately two months had started through heavy lifting as this is part of her job. The doctor could not help her except to give painkillers and the suggestion to take things easy.

She came to me and I examined her back thoroughly and found that there were no vertebrae out of place. I then proceeded to do Swiss Reflex Therapy with essential oils rather than back massage. The most tender spots were the lower back on both boot and the sciatic nerve affecting the hip. These areas were massaged on the feet for about fifteen minutes until they were hardly painful. I gave her a special oil to put into the bath mixed mainly with juniper and rosemary. Another appointment was made for the following week. The next day Miss C. was in a lot more pain in her back; the day after that the back was completely free from pain and stayed like that. When she came to me the following week she was completely pain free whereas before she had to miss work and was in tears because of the pain. I saw her recently six weeks after her last treatment and she was still pain free and had been able to go about her normal duties of work unhindered!

Mr C., a county cricket club captain, had not been able to bowl since the beginning of February, and it was now nearing the end of May. Everyone had said that he had neck trouble with not being able to twist his arm around for bowling; he also had terrible headaches. An osteopath, physiotherapist and acupuncturist had all been treating him since February for his neck.

On my first treatment of him I found that there were tender spots on his neck, head and also in his middle back (of which he was quite surprised). After this first treatment he found that his neck was much easier. I saw him for about three times a week over four weeks for about twenty minutes of Swiss Reflex Therapy with essential oils each time. At first he and the physiotherapist were puzzled that I kept finding a problem spot in the middle back. The physiotherapist had a more careful look down the back and found that there was a weakness in a disc in the middle back which was causing the neck and headache problems.

Slowly he started practising bowling as he felt fit. About five weeks after I had started treatment he bowled for the first time in a match and he did fantastically; the newspapers all commented on his performance.

If it had not been for SRT with essential oils the problem might never have been found and solved. Now the physiotherapist knows where to massage; rather than just concentrating on the neck he is mainly massaging the back and so far the problem has not returned.

One elderly woman came with osteoarthritis. Her right ankle was also badly damaged; it had been broken and was badly bruised, with no movement in it whatsoever. She also had a form of diabetes and was taking tablets for it. She came twice a week for fifteen minutes of SRT for a few weeks and eventually she was able to have longer treatments at longer intervals. Essential oils were also used made into bath oil and also body oil. Eventually one was found that helped immediately and that was a mixture of marjoram, rosemary and eucalyptus. The diet was also changed to acid-alkaline balanced.

There is now no bruise on her right ankle and it has a lot more movement. Her arthritis has been greatly improved and she feels very well inside. (Once, after one Swiss reflex treatment, she said that she felt like running, she felt so well!) Her diabetes has improved and she is now on reduced dosage of the tablets.

One of my clients, an elderly man, had advanced cancer of the bones and prostate gland. He also had arthritis and high blood pressure. He was taking drugs for the cancer and high blood pressure, plus 500mg of aspirin every day.

At first I did not know if I could do anything to help him and he understood this but was quite willing to have a try. I found through the foot reflex diagnostic technique that the whole body was out of balance, so I was very careful, treating for about ten minutes each time, on average twice a week. He dropped the aspirin straight away at commencement of the treatment. During three months of treatment he had stopped taking drugs for high blood pressure because the doctor had announced that it was now normal (it has stayed that way). He has never taken any aspirin since the start of the treatment.

Most of the tablets used to restrict his cancer have been stopped by the doctor. Generally his pain, although still there, is much improved; he used to walk with a walking stick which he does not need now. He has put on a lot of weight and looks quite sprightly and fit now. He is constantly improving as much as his age will allow.

There were other factors involved as well as the Swiss reflex treatment. An aromatherapy oil was made up for him to use at home to help his aches and pains and also a bath oil. His diet was also changed to acid-alkaline balanced. A very good multivitamin tablet, plus vitamin C (2gm daily) was also taken.

Another client came to me very nervous, tense but with no real medical problem. I decided that the best course of treatment would be aromatherapy treatments, so full aromatherapy was given using calming oils.

She felt much more relaxed for a long while afterwards, and now whenever she feels as though she is slipping back, immediately books for an aromatherapy massage.

One client regularly comes for aromatherapy treatments about every six weeks. She finds that the aromatherapy keeps all her aches and pains at bay for a few weeks, plus making her feel well inside. In between treatments she uses an aromatherapy bath oil which I make up, similar to that which she has in her treatment.

There is one woman I see once every so often when she feels depressed – from personal problems more than anything else. She just has SRT whenever she needs it, and I generally see her about once every three months.

From June Ronald:

Mrs A. had suffered from sinusitis for years and had tried various cures from her GP – medicines, sprays and more recently nasal syringes. She had experienced considerable relief after one aromatherapy treatment. Client was also given advice on how to use essential oils at home, and has since been feeling better than she has for years.

Miss B. had been suffering from insomnia for some years, and has been taking tranquillizers constantly. After one aromatherapy she slept regularly and soundly every night of the following week without drugs.

Miss C. was overweight though not obese. Excess weight was mainly in the form of cellulite. After a course of aromatherapy treatments the cellulite and hence her overall weight was considerably reduced.

Mrs D., aged 36, had failed to menstruate for six months though the pain continued, she felt depressed, and her weight increased. Advised by GP that this was due to menopause, her condition was diagnosed by aromatherapist as being due to a blockage, and after one aromatherapy treatment menstruation began the following day and associated problems quickly disappeared.

Miss E., aged 22, came for treatment three weeks before her wedding, unable to cope with pre-nuptial pressures. After two aromatherapy treatments the client felt and looked much better and was reported to be a 'radiant bride' on the big day.

Miss F. suffered from pain in her right side. Her GP was only able to prescribe pain killers. Aromatherapist diagnosed a kidney condition. The client was advised to drink plenty of water and after a few aromatherapy treatments the pain had abated considerably.

From Jackie Robertson and Brenda Etherington:

*Name:* Mrs L.
*Diagnosis:* Client suffers from extreme tension due to pressure of work, aches and muscular pains in lumbar region of back due to bending and lifting at work throughout the day. There is congestion in the back especially the lung area, due to heavy smoking. Client also suffers from cramp and an extremely dry skin, especially hands as they are always wet due to arranging flowers at work.
*Treatment:* The client came in at two week intervals and now comes in regularly every month.

*Oils used:* Juniper, lavender, sandalwood (avocado oil was added for quick penetration and for nourishment to skin).

*Result:* After the first treatment the client remarked that she felt as though a great weight had been lifted off her shoulders and head, and she felt very rested and relaxed. On her second visit she had been very busy at work putting in long hours and her whole body was aching. As I worked through the massage with more concentration on the knees and hands, she remarked that as I finished each particular part it ceased to ache. Client was given creams and oils for home use, mainly for dry skin and cramp; she has found a great improvement in general well-being and is more relaxed at work.

*Name:* Mrs M.

*Diagnosis:* Client was found to have bad circulation and congestion in lumbar region of back, mainly the right side where it was found that client suffers from arthritis in right hip. Due to the pain and discomfort of the arthritis the client was unable to get a restful night's sleep. The client is very fond of knitting and has knitted for many years for family and friends, and suffers from rheumatism in the joints of her hands, so being unable to knit for long. Client was also suffering from migraine headaches, found to be caused by the glasses she wore.

*Treatment:* Client came in each week for three weeks, and now comes in monthly.

*Oils used:* Eucalyptus, rosemary, sage.

*Result:* Client found great improvement in her general well-being and health. There was great ease in the right hip and client had much more restful nights and a great deal more movement of the whole right hip and leg. Knitting was much easier as the rheumatic pains in her hands had been alleviated. Client found that cold and damp weather affected her bad hip so a cream was made up for home use, and client has ceased to be bothered by her hip.

*Name:* Mr M.

*Diagnosis:* Client had given his left knee a knock, causing it to swell and causing discomfort and loss of movement. Client also suffered from pains all over his back but more so in the lumbar region, first thought to be due to work. But after a consultation with his doctor he was found to have 'Sherman's disease' for which there is no known cure. Client was very tense due to work and also the discomfort of his back. Client has suffered from sinus since childhood. Due to overnight travelling to work he was suffering from insomnia and eyestrain.

*Oils used:* Sage, juniper, lavender, jasmine.

*Result:* At the beginning of treatment the client was very tense and unable to relax, but after some gentle reassurance the client became so relaxed he could be moved like a puppet. There was found to be much ease in the back and the swelling in the knee went down. The client also found breathing much easier. The client was given oils and creams for home use; a bath oil and body lotion to use nightly for his back. He has found great ease, for the pain has been alleviated and he is able to work much better. He was also given a cream for his sinus problem and has found breathing easier.

# USEFUL ADDRESSES

## *AROMATOLOGY / AROMATHERAPY ASSOCIATIONS*

Institute of Aromatic Medicine
Aromed House
66 Upper Bond Street
Hinckley
Leics
LE10 1RS
Tel/Fax: 01455 611829

International Society of Professional Aromatherapists
ISPA House
82 Ashby Road
Hinckley
Leics
LE10 1SN
Tel: 01455 637987
Fax: 01455 890956

International Federation of Aromatherapists
Stamford House
2–4 Chiswick High Road
London
W4 1TH
Tel: 0181 742 2605

Register of Qualified Aromatherapists
PO Box 3431
Danbury
Chelmsford
Essex
CM3 4UA
Tel: 01245 227957

## SUPPLIES AND TRAINING

### Great Britain
Shirley Price Aromatherapy Ltd
Essentia House
Upper Bond Street
Hinckley
Leics
LE10 1RS
Tel: 01455 615466
Fax: 01455 615054

## *AROMATHERAPY TRAINING AND ESSENTIAL OILS*

### *Worldwide*

*Australia*

Margaret McGregor
Australian School of Awareness
PO Box 187
Montrose 3765
Australia
Tel: 00 61 397 618895
Fax: 00 61 397 288630

*Israel*

Fern Allen
PO Box 4363
Jerusalem, Israel
Tel: 00 972 2561 0043
Fax: 00 972 678 9908

*Italy*

Jenny Bird
Via Vigevano 43
Milan 20144
Italy
Tel: 00 39 258 113261

*Northern Ireland*

Mary Thompson
European College of Natural Therapies
16 North Parade
Belfast BT7 2GG
Tel: 01232 641454

*Norway*
Margareth Thomte
Nedreslottsgate 25
0157 Oslo
Norway
Tel: 00 47 22 170017
Fax: 00 47 22 425777

*Republic of Ireland*
Mary Cavanagh
Chamomile
Three Mile Cross
Wicklow
Eire
Tel: 00 353 404 47319

*Switzerland*
Sara Gelzer
Eigentalstr 552, No 14
8425 Oberembrach
Switzerland
Tel: 00 41 1865 4996

*USA*
Hans Nordblom
Nordblom Swedish Healthcare Centre
178 Mill Creek Road
Livingstone
Montana 59047
USA
Tel: 001 406 333 4216
Fax: 001 406 333 4415

## *SUPPLIERS OF SHIRLEY PRICE PRODUCTS*

*Great Britain*
Herbal Garden
20 Eldon Gardens
Percey Street
Newcastle upon Tyne
Tyne & Wear
NE1 7RA
Tel: 0191 230 3126

Herbal Garden
93 Rose Street
Edinburgh
Lothian
EH12 3DT
Tel: 0131 220 0251

*Northern Ireland*
Angela Hillis
32 Russell Park
Belfast
Co. Antrim
BT5 7QW

*Iceland*
Bergfell ehf
Skipholt 50c
105 Reykjavik, Iceland
Tel: 00 354 551 6690
Fax: 00 354 551 6956

*Japan*
Oz International Ltd
KS Building, 6F 4–5
Kojimachi
Chiyoda-Ku
Tokyo 102 003
Tel: 00 81 3 5213 3060
Fax: 00 81 3 3262 1970

*Korea*
Jung Dong Cosmetics Ltd
501 Shinham Officetel
49-5 Chungdam-Dong
Kangnam-Ku
Seoul, Korea

*Singapore*
Li & Low Marketing Pte Ltd
63 Hillview Avenue
09–21 Lam Soon Industrial Building
Singapore 2366
Tel: 00 65 7696168
Fax: 00 65 7693937

*Taiwan*
Jong Yeong Cosmetics Co Ltd
16 Tze Chyang 3rd Road
Nan Kang Industry Park
Nan Tou, Taiwan
Tel: 00 866 492 51065
Fax: 00 886 492 51071

# INDEX

abdomen massage 101-4
absolutes 7, 13, 74, 78, 120
acne 115
acupressure 5, 34, 39, 48
acupuncture 1, 33, 34, 46, 197, 205-6
additives 3
adulteration 133-4
ageing process 2
allergies 17, 18, 51, 52
allopathic drugs 32
almond oil 115
alphabetical list 136-7
alternative therapies 31, 38
animal fat 4
aniseed oil 154-5
anti-inflammatories 115, 117, 118
applied kinesiology 50-2
arm massage 111-12
aromatherapy
    essential oils 7-15
    massage explanation 82-6
    massage techniques 87-113
    recipes 120-32
    therapeutic index 182-96
    treatment techniques 73-81
arthritis 52, 80, 118
    case histories 199, 205, 210-11, 214-15
    recipes 127
assessment questions 61-2
asthma 17, 51, 76, 198, 199

aura healing 35
autonomic nervous system 44, 46
avocado oil 115, 116

back massage 87, 88-97
backache 32, 61, 209
base notes 11, 120, 122, 136-7, 170-81
basil oil 138-9
baths 5, 6, 37, 52
    case histories 202-3, 212
    recipes 120, 125-6
    treatment techniques 73, 77-8
benzoin oil 74, 170
bergamot oil 75, 139-40
black pepper oil 155-6
blending 87, 124, 126, 134-5, 138
blockages 55-8
blood circulation 1-2, 4, 56-7
    case histories 198
    massage 83, 85
    recipes 131
    SRT 59
blood pressure 129, 211
blue gum oil 143-4
body lotions 17, 22
breathing 60, 87
broken veins 18, 118
bronchitis 127, 208

cajuput oil 140-1

calendula oil 115, 117
cancer 211
caraway oil 141
carrier oils 87, 115-18
   case histories 204
   massage 126
   recipes 121-2, 125
   table 135
carrot oil 117
case histories 197-215
cedarwood oil 171
cell regeneration 2, 19, 20
cellulite 128, 199, 208, 213
chamomile oil 119, 156-7
chilblains 128
Chinese medicine 35
churches 36
circulatory system 34, 70, 78, 83
   case histories 206, 208, 214
   recipes 131
   therapeutic index 182
clary-sage oil 142-3
cleansers 17, 18, 23-6, 199
client participation 61-3
clove oil 171-2
coeliac plexus 46
cold pressed oils 115
cold sores 80
colds 128
colour healing 35
complementary therapies 31-52
compresses 5, 37, 73, 78-80, 86, 125-6
compression 43, 83-5
coniferae 9
constipation 204
coriander oil 143
corn oil 115, 116
cramp 128, 201-2, 213-14
crystal healing 35, 37
cucumber 23, 24, 25
cypress oil 157-8

depression 212
dermatitis 18, 129, 198
dermis 19, 20, 21

diabetes 210-11
diagnosis 37-8, 43, 46
   case histories 211
   SRT 52-3, 60, 62-72
diet 3-4, 16, 19, 31
   case histories 197, 201, 211
   holism 51-2
digestive system 4, 34, 44, 59
   case histories 206
   recipes 124, 129
   SRT 62-3, 68-9, 71
   therapeutic index 182-5
   treatment techniques 80
distillation 7, 8, 13-14, 74, 117, 133

ears 66
eczema 17, 18, 115, 117
   case histories 197-200, 203
   recipes 129
effects of oils 136-7
effleurage 83-4
embrocation 80
empathy 60
energy-based therapies 33-5
enfleurage 11-12
epidermis 18, 19
essential oils 3, 4-6, 7-15
   alphabetical list 136-7
   blending 87
   complementary therapies 36-7, 39, 51-2
   massage 114-19
   preparation 118-19
   recipes 120-32
   skin 17-18, 20
   SRT 53, 56
   table 120, 123, 133-81
   therapeutic index 182-96
   treatment techniques 73-81
eucalyptus oil 9, 135, 143-5
evaporation 10-11, 15, 21
evening primrose oil 115
excretory system 34, 59, 63, 68, 185-6
exercise 1, 4, 31
expression 11
eyes 22-5, 30, 66

face massage 104-11, 202
feedback 58
feelings 4
feet 22, 37, 43
    baths 77
    holism 47-50
    perspiring 131
    reflex points 55
fennel oil 119, 158-9
floral water 14
fluid retention 78, 200
France 37
frankincense oil 172-3
friar's balsam 170
frictions 83, 84-5

gargling 80
geranium oil 14, 124, 159-60
ginger oil 173
glandular system 34, 65
gout 196
grapeseed oil 115, 116

haemorrhoids 118
hair 16, 132, 203-4
hands 17, 22, 37, 43, 47, 77
harvesting 8
hay fever 17, 198, 199
hazelnut oil 115, 116
head 186-7
headaches 18, 76, 78, 202, 209-10, 214
herbal medicine 36
herpes 80
holism 31-52
homoeopathy 35
honey 75
hormones 4, 19, 196
hypericum oil 115, 117, 118
hypnosis 3, 32
hyssop oil 160-1

immune system 32-3, 196
indigestion 129, 206
ingestion 37, 74-6, 125
inhalations 5, 37, 73, 76, 125

insect repellent 129, 202
insomnia 18, 78, 129-30, 204, 212
involuntary reactions 44, 45
iridology 38

jasmine oil 14, 74, 120, 135, 174
jojoba 115
juniper oil 161-2

kidneys 69, 207-8, 213
kinesiology 35, 37, 50-2
Kirlian photography 33
kneading 83, 84

labour 32-3, 196
lamiaceae 9
lanolin 18, 20, 22-5
lavandin oil 162-3
lavender oil 9, 119-20, 163-4
leg massage 98-101, 113
lemon oil 124, 145-6
lemongrass oil 8, 146-7
lime blossom oil 117
lotions 118-19
lymphatic system 1-2, 5, 70, 83, 208

maceration 12, 117, 118, 126
marigold oil 117
marjoram oil 164-5
masks 17, 22-5, 27-8, 198
massage
    *see also* Swiss reflex therapy 5-6, 37, 74,
        125
    carrier oils 126
    case histories 212
    essential oils 114-19, 120-1
    explanation 82-6
    SRT 60-1
    techniques 87-113, 126
meditation 32
melissa oil 14, 117, 134-5, 165-6
menstruation 78, 80, 122
    case histories 201, 204, 213
    therapeutic index 188
meridian lines 33, 34, 40-3, 46, 50

middle notes 11, 120, 122
table 136-7, 154-70
midwifery 32
migraine 121-2, 130, 214
mind 2, 4
mind dynamics 3, 32
mineral oil 18-19, 23, 25, 114, 198
moisturizers 17-18, 21, 23-5, 29, 198, 203
multivitamins 211
muscular system 34, 66-7, 78-9, 130, 189
myrrh 174-5
myrtacae 9

naturopathy 197
neck reflex 67
neroli oil 120, 175-6
nervous system 34, 44-6, 64, 190-1
neuro-muscular technique 5
neuroses 206
New Age therapies 36
niaouli oil 147
night cream 17-18, 20-3, 25, 30, 200, 203
nutmeg oil 176-7

oil glands 20
olfactory nerves 6
olive oil 115, 117
orange blossom oil 120
orange oil 124, 135, 148
origanum oil 177-8

pain thresholds 61
palliative care 32
patchouli oil 178
peachnut oil 115
peppermint oil 10, 166-7
percussion 85
periods 122, 130, 188, 201, 204
petitgrain oil 149
petrissage 84
phytotherapy 36, 37
pine needle oil 167
pomades 12
positive thinking 32
postnatal depression 33

posture 1, 4
pregnancy 32, 86, 199
press point therapy 34, 43
professional associations 38-9, 216-17
psoriasis 17, 18, 115, 200-1

questions 62-3

rashes 201
recipes 120-32
reflexes 55, 58-9, 71-2
reflexology 33-5, 37-8, 43-50
    case histories 197
    massage 82
    SRT 52-4, 56
reproductive system 34, 70
resinoids 7, 13, 74, 78, 170
respiratory system 34, 61, 67, 191-2
rheumatism 115, 117-18
    case histories 202, 207
    recipes 121, 127, 130
rose oil 7, 9, 14, 74
    massage 119-20
    table 135, 179
rosehip oil 115
rosemary oil 134, 168-9
roughage 4

sage oil 119, 149-50
St John's wort oil 117, 118
sandalwood oil 14-15, 124, 180
savory oil 169-70
scalp 104, 186-7, 203-4, 206
scar tissue 86, 115, 199
sebum 20
self-application 80, 126
Sherman's disease 215
shiatsu 5, 33, 35, 37-43
    massage 82
    SRT 52
Shirley Price Aromatherapy 55, 118-19, 217
shoulders 112
showers 6
side effects 10, 17, 32, 37, 47, 134
sinuses 18, 66, 76

case histories 202-3, 212, 215
recipes 131
skeletal system 34
skin 16-30, 78-9, 117
    care routine 23-30
    case histories 198, 200, 203
    table 137
    therapeutic index 192-5
soap 16-19
solar plexus 46, 61, 64, 65
solvent extraction 12-13
soya bean oil 115
spine reflex 66
sprains 202
steam distillation 7, 13-14
steroids 17
storage 15, 116
stress 4, 16, 18, 31-2
    case histories 205
    holism 43
    recipes 120, 130
    SRT 57, 61
stretch marks 32, 127, 199
sugar 4, 51
sunburn 115
sunflower oil 115, 117
supplies 217, 218-21
sweat glands 20-1
Swiss Reflex Therapy (SRT) 50, 53-72
    case histories 207, 209-10
    treatment techniques 73
swollen ankles 32, 207
synergy 123

table of essential oils 120, 123, 133-81
tea tree oil 151

teas 75, 120, 124-6
tension 1-2, 4, 57
    case histories 206-7, 211-14
    recipes 120, 122, 131
    treatment techniques 76, 78
therapeutic index 79, 120, 121, 182-96
thumb frictions 82
thumb technique 50
thyme oil 10, 151-4
toners 17, 23, 25, 27
top notes 11, 120, 122, 136-7, 138-54
touch for health 50-2
training 217, 218-19
treatment techniques 73-81
tsubos 40

useful addresses 216-21

varicose veins 86, 118
vegetable oil 114-17, 126, 134
veruccas 196
virus infections 80
voluntary reactions 44

warts 196
wheatgerm oil 115, 116
wrinkles 22, 23

yang 35, 39-41
yin 35, 39-40, 42
ylang-ylang oil 8, 181
yoga 3, 32
yoghurt 23, 24, 25, 77

zone therapy 43
zones system 34